DATE DUE

Using Literature to Help
Troubled Teenagers
Cope with Identity Issues

Recent Titles in
The Greenwood Press "Using Literature to Help Troubled Teenagers"
Series

Using Literature to Help Troubled Teenagers Cope with Family Issues
Joan F. Kaywell, editor

Using Literature to Help Troubled Teenagers Cope with Societal Issues
Pamela S. Carroll, editor

Using Literature to Help Troubled Teenagers Cope with Identity Issues

Edited by
Jeffrey S. Kaplan

The Greenwood Press "Using Literature
to Help Troubled Teenagers" Series
Joan F. Kaywell, Series Adviser

Greenwood Press
Westport, Connecticut • London

Library of Congress Cataloging-in-Publication Data

Using literature to help troubled teenagers cope with identity issues
/ edited by Jeffrey S. Kaplan.
    p. cm.—(The Greenwood Press "Using literature to help
troubled teenagers" series)
  Includes bibliographical references and index.
  ISBN 0–313–30532–3 (alk. paper)
  1. Bibliotherapy for teenagers. 2. Identity (Psychology) in
adolescence. I. Kaplan, Jeffrey S., 1951– . II. Series.
RJ505.B5U844   1999
616.89'166'0835—dc21   99–21708

British Library Cataloguing in Publication Data is available.

Library of Congress Catalog Card Number: 99–21708
ISBN: 0–313–30532–3

First published in 1999

Greenwood Press, 88 Post Road West, Westport, CT 06881
An imprint of Greenwood Publishing Group, Inc.
www.greenwood.com

Printed in the United States of America

∞™

The paper used in this book complies with the
Permanent Paper Standard issued by the National
Information Standards Organization (Z39.48–1984).

10 9 8 7 6 5 4 3 2 1

**For my wife and daughter,
Renée and Lauren**

Contents

Series Foreword

The idea for this six-volume series—addressing family issues, identity issues, social issues, abuse issues, health issues, and death and dying issues—came while I, myself, was going to a therapist to help me deal with the loss of a loved one. My therapy revealed that I was a "severe trauma survivor" and I had to process the emotions of a bad period of time during my childhood. I was amazed that a trauma of my youth could be triggered by an emotional upset in my adult life. After an amazing breakthrough that occurred after extensive reading, writing, and talking, I looked at my therapist and said, "My God! I'm like the gifted child with the best teacher. What about all of those children who survive situations worse than mine and do not choose education as their escape of choice?" I began to wonder about the huge number of troubled teenagers who were not getting the professional treatment they needed. I pondered about those adolescents who were fortunate enough to get psychological treatment but were illiterate. Finally, I began to question if there were ways to help them while also improving their literacy development.

My thinking generated two theories on which this series is based: (1) Being literate increases a person's chances of emotional health, and (2) Twenty-five percent of today's students are "unteachable." The first theory was generated by my pondering these two statistics: 80% of our prisoners are illiterate (Hodgkinson, 1991), and 80% of our prisoners have been sexually abused (Child Abuse Council, 1993). If a correlation actually exists between these two statistics, then it suggests a strong need for literacy skills in order for a person to be able to address emotional turmoil in healthy or constructive ways. The second theory came out of work I did for my book, *Adolescents at Risk: A Guide to Fiction and Nonfiction for Young Adults, Parents and Professionals* (Greenwood Press, 1993), and my involvement in working with teachers and students in middle and secondary schools. Some of the emotional baggage our youth bring to school is way too heavy for them to handle without help. These students simply cannot handle additional academic responsibilities when they are "not right" emotionally.

THEORY ONE: BEING LITERATE INCREASES A PERSON'S CHANCES OF EMOTIONAL HEALTH

Well-educated adults who experience intense emotional pain, whether it is from the loss of a loved one or from a traumatic event, have several options available for dealing with their feelings. Most will find comfort in talking with friends or family members, and some will resort to reading books to find the help they need. For example, reading Dr. Elizabeth Kübler-Ross's five stages for coping with death—denial, anger, bargaining, depression, and acceptance or growth—might help a person understand the various stages he or she is going through after the death of a friend or relative. Sometimes, however, additional help is needed when an individual is experiencing extreme emotions and is unable to handle them.

Consider a mother whose improper left-hand turn causes the death of her seven-year-old daughter and the injury of her four-year-old daughter. It is quite probable that the mother will need to seek additional help from a therapist who will help her deal with such a trauma. A psychologist or psychiatrist will, more than likely, get her to talk openly about her feelings, read some books written by others who have survived such a tragedy, and do regular journal writing. A psychiatrist may also prescribe some medication during this emotionally challenging time. This parent's literacy skills of talking, reading, and writing are essential to her getting through this difficult period of her life.

Now, consider her four-year-old daughter who is also experiencing extreme grief over the loss of her beloved older sister. If this child is taken to counseling, the therapist will probably get her to talk, role-play, and draw out her feelings. These are the literacy skills appropriate to the developmental level of a four-year-old child. Such a child, if not taken to a counselor when needed, will manifest her emotions in one of two ways—either by acting out or by withdrawing.

Lev Vygotsky, a well-respected learning theorist, suggests that without words there could be no thoughts and the more words a person has at his or her disposal, the bigger that person's world. If what Vygotsky suggests is true, then a person with a limited or no vocabulary is only capable of operating at an emotional level. *The Story of My Life* by Helen Keller adds credibility to that view. In the introduction to the biography, written by Robert Russell, he describes Helen Keller's frustration at not being able to communicate:

> Perhaps the main cause for her early tantrums was plain frustration at not being able to communicate. . . . Not being able to hear, Helen had nothing to imitate, so she had no language. This meant more than simply not being able to talk. It meant having nothing clear to talk about because for her things had no names. Without names, things have no distinctness or individuality. Without language, we could not describe the difference between an elephant and an egg. Without the words we would have no clear conception of either elephant or egg. The name of a thing confers identity upon it and makes it possible for us to think about it. Without names for love or sorrow, we do not know we are experiencing them. Without words, we could not say, "I love you," and human beings need to say this and much more. Helen had the need, too, but she had not the means. As she grew older and the need increased, no wonder her fits of anger and misery grew. (pp. 7–9)

Helen, herself, writes,

> [T]he desire to express myself grew. The few signs I used became less and less adequate, and my failures to make myself understood were invariably followed by outbursts of passion. I felt as if invisible hands were holding me, and I made frantic efforts to free myself. I struggled—not that struggling helped matters, but the spirit of resistance was strong within me; I generally broke down in tears and physical exhaustion. If my mother happened to be near I crept into her arms, too miserable even to remember the cause of the tempest. After awhile the need of some means of communication became so urgent that these outbursts occurred daily, sometimes hourly. (p. 28)

If Vygotsky's theory reflected by the illuminating words of a deaf, blind, and mute child is true, then it is no wonder that 80% of our prisoners are illiterate victims of abuse.

THEORY TWO: 25% OF TODAY'S TEENAGERS ARE "UNTEACHABLE" BY TODAY'S STANDARDS

Teachers are finding it increasingly difficult to teach their students, and I believe that 25% of teenagers are "unteachable" by today's standards. A small percentage of these troubled youth do choose academics as their escape of choice, and they are the overachievers to the "nth" degree. That is not to say that all overachievers are emotionally disturbed teenagers, but some of them are learning, not because of their teachers, but because their very survival depends upon it. I know. I was one of them. The other adolescents going through inordinately difficult times (beyond the difficulty inherent in adolescence itself) might not find the curriculum very relevant to their lives. Their escapes of choice include rampant sex, drug use, gang membership, and other self-destructive behaviors. Perhaps the violence permeating our schools is a direct result of the utter frustration of some of our youth.

Consider these data describing the modern teenage family. At any given time, 25% of American children live with one parent, usually a divorced or never-married mother (Edwards & Young, 1992). Fifty percent of America's youth will spend some school years being raised by a single parent, and almost four million school-age children are being reared by neither parent (Hodgkinson, 1991). In 1990, 20% of American children grew up in poverty, and it is probable that 25% will be raised in poverty by the year 2000 (Howe, 1991). Children in homeless families often experience developmental delays, severe depression, anxiety, and learning disorders (Bassuk & Rubin, 1987).

Between one-fourth and one-third of school-aged children are living in a family with one or more alcoholics (Gress, 1988). Fourteen percent of children between the ages of 3 and 17 experience some form of family violence (Craig, 1992). Approximately 27% of girls and 16% of boys are sexually abused before the age of 18 (Krueger, 1993), and experts believe that it is reasonable to say that 25% of children will be sexually abused before adulthood (Child Abuse Council, 1993). Remember to note that eight out of ten criminals in prison were abused when they were children (Child Abuse Council, 1993).

Consider these data describing the modern teenager. Approximately two out of ten school-aged youth are affected by anorexia nervosa and bulimia (Phelps & Bajorek, 1991) and between 14% to 23% have vomited to lose weight (National Centers for Disease Control, 1991). By the time students become high school seniors, 90% have experimented with alcohol use and nearly two-thirds have used drugs (National Institute on Drug Abuse, 1992). In 1987, 40% of seniors admitted they had used dangerous drugs and 60% had used marijuana (National Adolescent Student Health Survey). In 1974, the average age American high school students tried marijuana was 16; in 1984, the average age was twelve (Nowinski, 1990).

By the age of 15, a fourth of the girls and a third of the boys are sexually active (Gibbs, 1993), and three out of four teenagers have had sexual intercourse by their senior year (Males, 1993). Seventy-five percent of the mothers who gave birth between the ages of 15 and 17 are on welfare (Simkins, 1984). In 1989, AIDS was the sixth leading cause of death for 15- to 24-year-olds (Tonks, 1992–1993), and many AIDS experts see adolescents as the third wave of individuals affected by HIV (Kaywell, 1993). Thirty-nine percent of sexually active teenagers said they preferred not to use any method of contraception (Harris Planned Parenthood Poll, 1986).

Ten percent of our students are gay (Williams, 1993), and the suicide rate for gay and lesbian teenagers is two to six times higher than that of heterosexual teens (Krueger, 1993). Suicide is the second leading cause of teenage deaths; "accidents" rated first (National Centers for Disease Control, 1987). An adolescent commits suicide every one hour and 47 minutes (National Center for Health Statistics, 1987), and nine children die from gunshot wounds every day in America (Edelman, 1989). For those children growing up in poor, high crime neighborhoods, one in three has seen a homicide by the time they reach adolescence (Beck, 1992).

Consider these data describing the dropout problem. In 1988, the dropout rate among high school students was 28.9% (Monroe, Borzi, & Burrell, 1992). More than 80% of America's one million prisoners are high school dropouts (Hodgkinson, 1991). We spend more than $20,000 per year per prisoner (Hodgkinson, 1991) but spend less than $4,000 per year per student. Forty-five percent of special education students drop out of high school (Wagner, 1989).

Numbers and statistics such as these are often incomprehensible, but consider the data in light of a 12th grade classroom of 30 students. Eight to 15 are being raised by a single parent, six are in poverty, eight to ten are being raised in families with alcoholics, four have experienced some form of family violence, and eight of the female and five of the male students have been sexually violated. Six are anorectic or bulimic, 27 have used alcohol, 18 have used marijuana, and 12 have used dangerous drugs. Twenty-two have had sexual intercourse and 12 of them used no protection. Three students are gay. Eight will drop out of school, and six of those eight will become criminals. Everyday in our country, two adolescents commit suicide by lunchtime.

These are the students that our teachers must teach every day, and these are the students who need help beyond what schools are currently able to provide. Think about the young adults who are both illiterate and in pain! Is there anything that can be done to help these young people with their problems while increasing their literacy skills? Since most of our nation's prisoners are illiterate—the acting out side—and most homeless people are not exactly Rhodes scholars—the withdrawal side— it seems logical to try to help these adolescents while they are still within the educational system.

Perhaps this series, which actually pairs literacy experts with therapists, can help the caretakers of our nation's distraught youth—teachers, counselors, parents, clergy, and librarians—acquire understanding and knowledge on how to better help these troubled teenagers. The series provides a unique approach to guide these caretakers working with troubled teenagers. Experts discuss young adult literature, while therapists provide analysis and advice for protagonists in these novels. Annotated bibliographies provide the reader with similar sources that can be used to help teenagers discuss these issues while increasing their literacy skills.

Joan F. Kaywell

REFERENCES

Bassuk, E. L. & Rubin, L. (1987). Homeless children: A neglected population. *American Journal of Orthopsychiatry, 57* (2), p. 279 ff.

Beck, J. (1992, May 19). Inner-city kids beat the odds to survive. *The Tampa Tribune.*

Craig, S. E. (1992, September). The educational needs of children living with violence. *Phi Delta Kappan, 74* (1), p. 67 ff.

Edelman, M. W. (1989, May). Defending America's children. *Educational Leadership, 46* (8), p. 77 ff.

Edwards, P. A. & Young, L. S. J. (1992, September). Beyond parents: Family, community, and school involvement. *Phi Delta Kappan, 74* (1), p. 72 ff.

Gibbs, N. (1993, May 24). How should we teach our children about sex? *Time, 140* (21), p. 60 ff.

Gress, J. R. (1988, March). Alcoholism's hidden curriculum. *Educational Leadership, 45* (6), p. 18 ff.

Hodgkinson, H. (1991, September). Reform versus reality. *Phi Delta Kappan, 73* (1), p. 9 ff.

Howe II, H. (1991, November). America 2000: A bumpy ride on four trains. *Phi Delta Kappan, 73* (3), p. 192 ff.

Kaywell, J. F. (1993). *Adolescents at risk: A guide to fiction and nonfiction for young adults, parents and professionals*. Westport, CT: Greenwood Press.

Keller, H. (1967). *The story of my life*. New York: Scholastic.

Krueger, M. M. (1993, March). Everyone is an exception: Assumptions to avoid in the sex education classroom. *Phi Delta Kappan, 74* (7), p. 569 ff.

Males, M. (1993, March). Schools, society, and "teen" pregnancy. *Phi Delta Kappan, 74* (7), p. 566 ff.

Monroe, C., Borzi, M. G., & Burrell, R. D. (1992, January). Communication apprehension among high school dropouts. *The School Counselor, 39* (4), p. 273 ff.

Nowinski, J. (1990). *Substance abuse in adolescents and young adults*. New York: Norton.

Phelps, L. & Bajorek, E. (1991). Eating disorders of the adolescent: Current issues in etiology, assessment, and treatment. *School Psychology Review, 20* (1), p. 9 ff.

Simkins, L. (1984, spring). Consequences of teenage pregnancy and motherhood. *Adolescence, 19* (73), p. 39 ff.

Tonks, D. (1992–1993, December–January). Can you save your students' lives? Educating to prevent AIDS. *Educational Leadership, 50* (4), p. 48 ff.

Wagner, M. (1989). *Youth with disabilities during transition: An overview of descriptive findings from the national longitudinal transition study*. Stanford, CA: SRI International.

Williams, R. F. (1993, spring). Gay and lesbian teenagers: A reading ladder for students, media specialists, and parents. *The ALAN Review, 20* (3), p. 12 ff.

Introduction

THE SEARCH FOR IDENTITY

When Joan Kaywell approached me with the invitation to edit one of the six volumes in this series, I jumped at the chance immediately. Here was a splendid opportunity for me to blend my many interests—literature, teenagers, and psychology. Although I am not a student of psychology, I am a huge fan of "adolescent thinking" and how that peculiar brand of individual manages to make their way in the world. As a public school teacher for some ten years, and now a university professor, I have learned to look at teenagers as both a subject and an object. While I taught school in many counties in Florida, the youngsters I encountered were like teenagers everywhere—energetic, lazy, happy, sad, optimistic, confused, and just plain goofy. They were the kids who populated my English and drama classes, and became the daily wonders of my amusement and consternation. "Why is your notebook such a mess?" "Why do you write one day with your left hand and the next day with your right?" "Why do you always wear black clothing?" "Why do you only listen to that rock group?" "Why do you always giggle?" "Why don't you ever eat your lunch?" "And why, oh why, are you so quiet in class? What are you thinking?"

To be sure, they were perplexing creatures, silly and wise all at once. Yet, as I began to teach education courses on the university level, I began to see them more in a clinical light. They became objects of my professorial lens, and their many shapes and configurations became more defined as I studied them, in person and on paper, in an even sharper light. Their goofiness became the subject of study, and when I began to familiarize myself with the works of eminent psychologists like Erikson, Kohlberg, Maslow, and Rogers, I began to realize that the "inherent craziness" of teenagers is just a manifestation of their search for themselves. Their struggle to define who they are and to bring forth their true identities became, for me, a fascinating journey toward understanding not only them, but myself.

As every parent knows, the teenage years are not an easy time. Dating, driving, and drinking (or not drinking) become the hallmarks of every family's discussions, and the "do's and don'ts" of proper behavior and decorum underlie a teenager's every move. Parents fret that they have not done enough to ensure their child's growth and success; teachers worry that they are not preparing their students for their next grade or career move; and teenagers agonize over every step because, for them, every step is their first step. The first time they kiss someone good night, or maybe hello. The first time they take the steering wheel of a car and leave the driveway. The first time they encounter religious or racial hostility and are left confused and angry. The first time they realize that their weight or height might make a difference in their appearance and they struggle to perfect themselves, or maybe hide. The first time they turn their back on their parents, asserting their own independence and their right to say no. The first time they feel totally different from their peers and look for some group or peer to lead the way. And the first time they shout from the rooftop of their souls, "I am different. I am me!"

As a theater major, I am aware of how important dramatics can be in teenagers' lives: the clothing they wear; the makeup they apply; the sayings they echo; the stance they take; the anger they express; the emotions they write; the pain they feel. All these things are manifestations of their search for who they really are, apart from parents, siblings, and friends, and their sincere, if often ill-fated, attempt to become who they hope to be. The quest is often painful and tortured, and not one any adult would care to repeat, but it is something we all must endure. Yet, how better to endure this pain than with a friend, and often, this friend can be a book.

WHY THIS BOOK?

This volume is designed for educators, therapists, parents, and others who want to know more about kids and growing up. The idea is to pair an educator who works with adolescents with a therapist (a psychologist, social worker, etc.) to look at a young adult novel from both a literary and a clinical perspective. The analysis is intended to be informative both for people who want to know more about the work as a literary creation and for those who want to know what noted therapists and social workers might prescribe to help the lead characters in the novel. It is as if the lead characters in these young adult novels were really alive and their problems could be solved by clinical practitioners.

Now, this might sound far-fetched because no literary character could ever duplicate the depth and breadth of a real person. But the chance to speculate on what might be, for the edification of all involved, is too tantalizing to resist. Besides, teenagers always turn to art—television, music, film, and often books—to find approximations of their own lives. So what better way to look at their problems than through the magic of well-told stories? And pairing educators with therapists allows these two types of specialists to exchange expertise and, thereby, to further illuminate the works in question. Finally, since adolescence is marked by the storm and stress of the never-ending quest for self-understanding, studying identity issues as they relate to young adult literature is most appropriate.

Adolescents, those gangly creatures from age 13 to 19, are on a constant search to define themselves. They look everywhere—in malls, at the movies, in school hallways, and at after-school teenage hangouts—to assert their independence and define their presence. Their search for who they are is universal, but unique to each individual. And no matter how many times they look, they often fall short. One day, they stumble unexpectedly upon someone just like them. And then—bingo! Almost as if manna has fallen from heaven, they begin to feel comfortable in their own skin. This quest to define their true selves is what is defined in each of the chapters in this book.

HOW WERE THE TOPICS CHOSEN?

Each of the contributors to this volume, teachers and therapists alike, has spent time with kids. Some are teachers who have logged in many years in classrooms across this country and elsewhere, working with young people as they taught them the "three Rs" and the "three Ss" (security, sincerity, and self-esteem). Now, many are university educators, and their desire to impart knowledge to future teachers about teaching literature or general academics to young people remains just as strong. Their ability to distill years of practical and academic learning into these few pages is a powerful testament to their ability to discern the truths about growing up. Other contributors are therapists who have much training in analyzing young adults, and the unique perspective of these specialists brings new light to some familiar, and some not-so-familiar, literary works. Their desire for the truth takes them on a journey that usually remains behind closed doors, and I am delighted that they have shared their insights in contributing to this book.

The young adult novels that are discussed in this volume were chosen by the contributors. The only stipulation was that the work, in keeping with the series, had to be a young adult novel. A young adult novel is a novel in which the protagonist is a teenager and the world is seen through a teenager's eyes. Often written in a vernacular that is popular among young adults, the work is best defined by a desire to see the world through a kid's eyes but still maintain the sophistication of an adult genre. Hence, many adults return to young adult novels—J. D. Salinger's *The Catcher in the Rye*, Robert Cormier's *The Chocolate War*, S. E. Hinton's *The Outsiders*, and Paul Zindel's *The Pigman*—when they desire to reread something for both pleasure and insight. "Now that I am older, maybe I will see something new."

Each chapter is arranged in a format appropriate to the topic at hand. Some give complete, straightforward descriptions of the work in question, followed by a clinical description of the leading characters in the novel. The educators discuss the literary merit of the work; the therapists explore the protagonist's motivation. Other chapters have a more conversational tone; the contributors let you "listen in" on their banter about plot, character, and desires, in the hope that the free-flowing question-and-answer format will prove to be both inviting and illuminating. In still others, contributors describe personal experiences, believing that their self-revelations will clarify the choices made by their fictional counterparts.

And although the chapters are slightly different in structure and tone, they all contain certain basic elements. Each chapter begins with a discussion of plot followed by an analysis of the novel's characters and a proposed therapy for them. The chapters conclude with an annotated list of recommended readings to help teens and those working with them find appropriate material that deals with their problems.

Finally, I asked Joan Bauer, a noted young adult novelist, to include her hilarious and poignant tale of how she—a white, middle-class, suburban adult—was invited to speak before a group of inner-city high school students about the joy of writing. Not surprisingly, the task was difficult, and she describes the frustration, and eventual satisfaction, she felt when she crossed this cultural divide. She relates how, although she and her audiences were miles apart economically and socially, she managed to find a common bond of friendship and struggle when she spoke openly about her own fears as a kid growing up and about her own special search for self.

A PERSONAL JOURNEY

Editors know they learn more than any contributor or reader. They spend more time with each individual entry and, of course, see the whole before the others see the individual sections. The thrust to cover all the bases—personal, social, and moral concerns—is always present, and the often painstaking task of deciding what good stuff to leave out, for the sake of time, money, or just plain space, can be agonizing to say the least. But, when it is done, the feeling of satisfaction can be overwhelming, and the pride in a job well done can put to rest any fears.

I love working with young adults because I learn so much when I ask questions. "What do you like to do after school?" "What is your home life like?" "What sports do you play?" "What music do you listen to?" "What makes you special?" "What books do you read?" This last question is often the most illuminating, for many young adults are unaware of the considerable number of good books available for teenagers. Frequently, wise and caring adults, such as parents, teachers, and therapists, can recommend good books for kids to read, to help them explore new universes and revisit old ones. This quest for self-knowledge is at the heart of any journey.

ACKNOWLEDGMENTS

The writing of a book is the collaboration of many people. First, I want to thank Emily Birch, Editor, at Greenwood Press, for her patience, care, and smart eye in preparing this manuscript, and naturally, the many fine contributors whose writing appears in the chapters that follow. Second, I want to thank my two mentors, Dr. Joan Kaywell, University of South Florida, Tampa, for her invitation to edit a volume in her original series, and Dr. Ted Hipple, University of Tennessee, Knoxville, for his expertise, friendship, and advice. Third, I want to thank Dr. Karen Biraimah, University of Central Florida, Orlando, for encouraging my efforts, and Ms. Hope Baril, University of Central Florida, Daytona Beach, for her profound support and humor. And finally, my parents, Anita and James Kaplan, and my wife and daughter, Renée and Lauren, for their love and devotion.

Prologue

Joan Bauer

I'm still not sure how the misunderstanding happened, but it was clear there had been a big one as I walked across the littered high school campus in Southern California and had to face the cold reality that the one-hour speech I had prepared for this ninth-grade assembly was wrong. All wrong.

I accepted the invitation from a friend of a friend of a friend, and somewhere along the line, there had been a miscommunication about the kind of school where I would be speaking. I thought it was a middle- to upper-middle-class high school and prepared accordingly—putting together a speech about writing from the heart and how characters and story lines are developed.

The teacher walking with me filled me in on the realities: Ninety-five percent of the student body had English as a second language. Very few of the four hundred ninth graders I would be addressing could read or write. So much for an in-depth discussion on writing styles and character development.

The teacher said she was a bit concerned about my speaking to such a large crowd of students because en masse these kids were rowdy.

"Define rowdy," I said. She smiled and unlocked a chain link fence. I followed her into the auditorium, past graffiti from rival street gangs.

What, I asked myself, could I possibly say to these kids that would connect us and make a difference? My mind was blank.

I stood by the podium, clutching my meaningless notes as the students swaggered in. They smelled blood. The janitor locked the door as a few boys looked me over and sneered.

"Hey, lady, you a writer? Write something about me 'cause I've had a bad, evil life."

"You don't look like a writer. Are you rich?"

"Only in spirit," I muttered.

"How come I never heard of you?"

I wish I could say that I immediately connected to these young people, that I quickly built a bridge of understanding between us. But the raw truth is that for what seemed like a lifetime, I bombed. Big time.

I couldn't find a place to begin. I tried talking about writing, but that didn't work. They weren't writers.

I tried talking about reading, but they couldn't care less about that.

They looked at me, and I looked at them, and the moat between us seemed too vast to ever cross. And I wondered if it was true, if I really had nothing to say to them.

Then somewhere deep within, I sensed an instinct. I went with it, grabbed a hand mike, and walked to the front row.

"Why," I half-shouted, "do you think stories are important?"

"They're not!" a boy cried from the back, and the room burst into laughter.

"Why not?" I asked him with much more confidence than I felt. He shrugged, looked away.

A girl raised her hand. "I like stories. I just don't like reading."

"What do you like about them?"

"They teach me things."

"They're fun," said another.

Entertainment and truth. We were onto something. I'm not sure how it happened, but I found myself telling them about the difficult time I had growing up with an alcoholic father. I told them how humor had helped me laugh at difficult things and helped me look at life in a more positive way because if I wasn't going to laugh, it was a safe bet I was going to cry. I told them that in the stories I wrote, I was trying to work things out, trying to make sense of the world in a humorous way, but still with seriousness.

I read to them from my novel *Squashed*—the scene at the mother's grave. I told them how I'd pulled the emotions for writing that scene from my own father's death. I shared with them what it was like for me to go back and visit his grave and feel the pain of his death all over again. Then a few hands went up, and kids were talking about uncles being shot, and sisters who were unmarried and pregnant, and all the lousy things that happen to people in a world we'd all like to be fair and safe but that isn't in so many places.

Then I told them that they knew more about writing and stories than they realized because the source of good storytelling and writing is emotion, often pain. They nodded. They knew about pain. I told them what Mark Twain said about humor: "The secret ingredient in humor isn't joy, but pain." They understood that at a very deep level.

I actually got to talk a little about character development. I read to them again. They loved being read to. We had a good question-and-answer session, and when it was over, I realized what a gift that hour had been to me. I'd seen the power of a story break down walls and build bridges. I'd learned firsthand how much we human beings have in common. I'd seen that kids are desperate to laugh and communicate and share. Young people are hungry for stories—not just for the entertainment stories provide, but because stories give voice to the silence, misunderstandings, adversities, and triumphs in their lives.

May they gobble up this book.

CHAPTER 1

Identity within the Family: Phyllis Reynolds Naylor's *The Year of the Gopher*

Lois T. Stover and J. Roy Hopkins

INTRODUCTION AND SYNOPSIS

"Who am I?" That is a question with which young adults wrestle throughout their teenage years. They try to find answers by examining their role within their family, rethinking their relationships with their friends, considering their sexual impulses, exploring career options, and investigating their values and beliefs. They test out various combinations of possibilities in a whirl of activity that makes them seem confused and rebellious to their parents and other significant adults in their lives. When Phyllis Reynolds Naylor's *The Year of the Gopher* (hereafter cited as *Gopher*) opens, George Richards, age 17, is in the midst of determining what he will do after he completes his senior year and graduates from high school. A good student, and generally a "good guy," George has not spent a great deal of time contemplating his options up to this point in his life. When confronted with the reality of his parents' expectations for his future, he begins to rebel, eventually taking a year off from school to work as a "gofer." He uses this year to think about what he wants for his future and learns a great deal about himself; he also teaches his parents some important lessons at the same time. Naylor's novel can serve as a useful backdrop against which to discuss important issues related to the process of answering the question "Who am I?" It also provides a useful case study of Erik Erikson's psychosocial theory of identity development.

George is the second of four children, and the oldest boy in the Richards family. As the eldest son, George has lived for seventeen years with the expectation that he will attend an Ivy League college, go on to law school, and become an attorney like his father and his grandfather before him. But during his senior year of high school, when the novel opens, George begins to question this vision of his future. When his father arranges to take a week off from his Minnesota legal practice and escort George on a tour of various East Coast colleges, George's disquiet becomes more pronounced. He is not certain what he wants to do, does not fully comprehend how he is feeling about himself, his future, and his role within his family, but he knows something is wrong. He doesn't feel he can explain himself to his father.

George begins to observe more closely the ways in which his parents interact with his younger brother and sister. Ollie, the youngest son, finds school difficult. Abstract academic content means little to him, and he has trouble learning new material. George understands that Ollie's talents lie in other areas, and George becomes very upset when he realizes his parents mistake Ollie's poor grades for a lack of caring and an unwillingness to stick with difficult tasks. As Mrs. Richards begins to catalog all the times when Ollie has given up on an activity, from clarinet lessons to scouting, George realizes that these projects had been selected *for*, not *by*, Ollie. As he reflects on Ollie's experiences as a Boy Scout, George begins to understand that while Ollie wanted to join the organization because of his love for camping and being outdoors, Mr. Richards assumed that being a scout meant striving, at a fast pace, to be an Eagle Scout. George reflects, "You couldn't just be a Scout in our family; you had to be the best there *was*" (*Gopher*, p. 59).

Applying this new insight to his own situation, George understands that his parents seem to need successful children in order to demonstrate their own success as parents. They measure their own accomplishments as mother and father through the awards and accomplishments of their children. And he begins to see that his parents experienced the same sort of pressures, especially his father, who had succumbed to his own father's need for a successful son. Therefore, George decides that he needs to derail the train on which he and his siblings are riding into the future. He decides to sabotage the college application process.

When the rejections begin to arrive, Mrs. Richards figures out what George has done. Confronting him, she asks him why he didn't just tell her what he was feeling. George almost shouts at her,

> I said it every way I knew how, but you weren't listening. . . . You don't care about me, you don't care about my education, you only care how it

makes you *look*. . . . Somebody had to make the break. I'm not going to end up at an Ivy League school with a bottle of Maalox just to please you and Dad. (*Gopher*, pp. 75–76)

And so begins "the year of the gopher." George continues to live at home, first taking a job doing manual labor and some sales clerking at a garden center, and then becoming a "gofer," riding a bike to make deliveries around the city. Naylor's skill at character development allows the reader to watch as George slowly gains a sense of self and a set of values on which he can base a future that makes sense to him, given his growing sense of his own skills and goals. As George interacts with the people in his life, he learns from those encounters. When the novel opens, he is merely rebellious and rather self-centered, but he moves toward self-awareness and develops a substantive core of beliefs that eventually allow him to make a career choice and, at the same time, to make a different kind of place for himself within his family.

One of Naylor's strengths as a novelist is that she juxtaposes characters. George learns a good deal about his own parents by contrasting them with Shirl, a clerk at the garden center where he lands his first job after high school graduation. Shirl is the mother of a young girl, Heather, for whom she has different, but still very definite, expectations. As George interacts with Heather, his decision to break with his parents is strengthened, and he begins to learn that he has some skill in working with young people. He begins to consider a career as a school guidance counselor.

Additionally, Naylor is able to make George's slow transformation into an independent young adult believable because she shows the reader the seeds of George's future self in his early actions. Therefore, his decision by the end of the novel to matriculate at the local university and pursue the goal of becoming a guidance counselor rings true because, as Steve Matthews writes in *School Library Journal*, Naylor "stops short of patness and reaffirms the complexity and pain of coming of age" (116). For instance, although George is definitely driven by hormones, concerned about his looks, influenced by his friends, and feeling rebellious toward his parents, even early in the story he is shown to be a young man with many redeeming characteristics. As Naylor gives us these glimpses of George's personality and strengths, she creates plot tensions and makes the reader appreciate just how little his parents know about their son.

George's willingness to take a stand, to grow, and to base his future on his developing value structure provide the core of the novel's plot.

Very early in the story, the reader meets Karen, in George's eyes the most beautiful girl in the school. He is upset to learn from his friend Jake, who works in a pharmacy, that Karen has purchased birth control pills; he knows exactly how the insensitive Jake must have smirked and teased Karen during the exchange. George describes how he might have handled such a transaction—in just a routine way, talking about school all the while—and he thinks how she would have appreciated the privacy involved (*Gopher*, p. 11). Naylor shows the reader, through George's actions, that he has a compassionate streak and an ability to see the world from another's point of view, which should serve him well in the world.

The reader believes George's discomfort when he falls into a sexual relationship with Maureen, a girl from his senior class who has actively pursued him for several years. He takes her to the prom, follows her suggestion that they go to the cemetery for a picnic afterward, and again follows her lead when she moves them into a more intimate relationship. Although he is not above bragging to his friends about his new set of sexual experiences, he is bothered by the casualness of the relationship. As he gains confidence and skill in expressing his values, he is able to tell Maureen that they need to say good-bye. He learns from his experiences with Maureen, so that when he meets a girl to whom he is genuinely attracted, he moves more slowly, working on getting to know her and on letting her know him, on becoming friends as a first step.

George is also uncomfortable with his parents' mandate that he stay out of the home of his friend Dave Hahn. Mr. and Mrs. Richards are horrified when they learn that Dave's father is bisexual, and they forbid George to have anything to do with Mr. Hahn. But George gradually comes to see that Mr. Hahn is just an average person struggling to make a place for himself in the world, and out of friendship for Dave, George spends time at the Hahn home, playing poker with father and son, coming to accept Mr. Hahn for who he is. George also becomes uncomfortable with the way in which his parents try to make decisions for his grandfather. Again, as he gains confidence, he argues on his grandfather's behalf that he be allowed to retain control over his own life.

George's decisions, predictably, cause chaos in the formerly smooth-running Richards household. Conversation comes to a halt; the parents and George speak in mere formalities, asking for the salt or acknowledging a phone message that has been passed along. But George's refusal to be rushed into college, to take the route into the future mapped out by his parents, creates enough disequilibrium for his mother that she, too, begins to question her own career path.

George's father is slower to come to terms with what he perceives as George's betrayal. Yet George gradually wins his father's respect. He does not complain about the difficulties of his various jobs. He budgets his time and money effectively. He carries out his commitments. By Christmas of the year after graduation, George's dad offers him a unique gift: a new bicycle, one better suited to the demands of a "gofer" riding through the city streets during a Midwestern winter. George knows how difficult it must have been for his dad to purchase that bike: "he was offering acceptance of who I was" (*Gopher*, p. 200). Buying the bike indicates just how far his father has come from the times when he would leave George a list from the business section of the paper of the income levels of various professions, with "Just thought you'd find this interesting" scribbled in the margins (*Gopher*, p. 21).

The Year of the Gopher provides, in George, a model for young people of how to move away from one's family in a positive way, and of how to use empathy and one's developing awareness of self and personal values as a basis for action.

ERIKSON'S THEORY OF IDENTITY

Erik Homburger Erikson (1902–1994) worked within the psychoanalytic tradition begun by Sigmund Freud in turn-of-the-century Vienna. However, Erikson significantly modified the Freudian approach to personality development, which had emphasized the importance of sexuality, particularly as it developed in early childhood, in determining the outcome of adult personality. Erikson's approach placed much greater emphasis on social interaction and has come to be called a "psychosocial" theory of development.

Two features set Erikson's psychosocial theory of identity development apart from other theories. First, his theory is epigenetic. This term, borrowed from embryology, means that there is an underlying blueprint for development that characterizes all human personality growth. We each have human potentialities, and we each experience particular types of interaction, such as being parented, being educated, coming to terms with sexuality, and so forth. As Erikson (1968) put it, the epigenetic principle "states that anything that grows has a ground plan, and that out of this ground plan the parts arise, each part having its time of special ascendancy, until all parts have arisen to form a functioning whole" (92). That functioning whole is the individual personality, and as we all know, there is great variety in individual human personalities. But there is regularity in the ways that we come to develop our individuality, as we move from the somewhat sheltered sphere of the nuclear family, to the larger environment of schools, to the rich tapestry of individual occupations available in adulthood. Erikson elaborated further on the epigenetic principle:

> [I]t is important to realize that in the sequence of his most personal experiences the healthy child, given a reasonable amount of proper guidance, can be trusted to obey inner laws of development, laws which create a succession of potentialities for significant interaction with those persons who tend and respond to him and those institutions which are ready for him. (93)

The second feature that sets Erikson's theory apart, which is also linked to the concept of epigenesis, is that each stage of personality development has its characteristic "normative crisis"—a time of heightened vulnerability and potential for growth. When Erikson says that each part of the ground plan has "its time of special ascendancy," he means that there is a stage of development during which that feature of personality is especially prominent.

In Erikson's model, there are eight stages of development in the life cycle, each with its own normative crisis. The first three stages are centered around social interaction within the nuclear family: trust vs. mistrust in infancy; autonomy vs. shame and doubt in toddlerhood; and initiative vs. guilt in early childhood. As the child's social sphere widens in childhood, particularly with entry into formal schooling, the child enters the stage of industry vs. inferiority, which lasts until about puberty. The physical changes of puberty form the rough demarcation point for entering adolescence, a stage of intense self-focus. The normative crisis for this key stage is identity vs. role confusion. The three phases of adulthood in Erikson's life-cycle theory are: intimacy vs. isolation in early adulthood; generativity vs. stagnation, the longest stage, associated with middle adulthood; and ego integrity vs. despair, the stage of late adulthood.

ERIKSON'S STAGES AND THE RICHARDS FAMILY

In *The Year of the Gopher*, key characters represent several of these life stages. George Richards, the central character, is clearly in the stage of identity vs. role confusion. George's younger sister, Jeri, is also in this stage. Younger brother Ollie is at the end of the stage of industry vs. inferiority. Older sister Trish is in the stage of intimacy vs. isolation, but she also illustrates some of the gender politics of identity, which link identity and intimacy for many young women. George's parents are in the generativity vs. stagnation stage, and his grandfather is in the ego integrity vs. despair stage.

Identity Statuses in Adolescence

An identity "crisis" is not a debilitating personal tragedy, as some might think, but rather a period of heightened vulnerability about the self. It usually involves some fairly intense exploration of various elements of identity—occupational decision making, ideologies of various types (such as religious, political, and sexual), and so on. The exploration of identity inherent in this normative crisis can make adolescence appear flighty and fickle, as various roles are tried out and discarded. Psychologically, in Erikson's theoretical model, the exploration carries great importance for personality development. As the stage of adolescence draws to a close, the individual begins to make important commitments, to occupation, to sexual role, to political and religious ideology. These commitments are not fixed in stone, but at the same time they are no longer as fluid as they were before the normative crisis of identity vs. role confusion.

Several researchers (Balistreri, Busch-Rossnagel, and Geisinger, 1995; Marcia, 1983; Rugow, Marcia, and Slugoski, 1983; Schiedel and Marcia, 1985; Slugoski, Marcia, and Koopman, 1984) have examined Erikson's notion of crisis and commitment in adolescence by interviewing adolescents about their experiences or by using questionnaires to gauge their level of exploration and commitment in various areas. Most notable among these researchers is James Marcia. Marcia (1966) proposed four identity statuses. Adolescents who have not experienced the intense exploration associated with the identity crisis and who have made no real commitments, are said to be in "role confusion." Some individuals go through the entire period of adolescence in role confusion and may be said to "resolve" this normative crisis with a sense of role confusion or identity diffusion.

Those adolescents who have not experienced any real identity exploration, but who have nevertheless made commitments, are said to be in "identity foreclosure"; they have committed to something, such as a career path, before they are ready for it. Adolescents who are experiencing identity exploration, but still have not made any commitments, are in a status called a "psychosocial moratorium." Such a moratorium, according to Erikson, is a good thing, provided it does not go on for too long. To successfully resolve the normative crisis of adolescence, one needs both the exploration and the commitment. The identity status associated with both exploration and commitment is "identity achievement."

Occupational Identity Status in The Year of the Gopher

George lets us know very early in *The Year of the Gopher* that his parents are pressuring him into a career path that he does not want. In fact, as the novel begins, George has no idea what he wants to do. But his parents want him to apply to an Ivy League college, as we learn on the novel's first page, when the Dartmouth and Princeton catalogs arrive "kerplunk" through the mail slot. One of the most forceful reasons that adolescents adopt an identity status of foreclosure is parental pressure. Parents often try to make decisions for their adolescent children, particularly about choosing a career path. This pressure is very difficult to resist, especially in young people who want very much to please their parents, or who feel obligated to follow the wishes of their parents because they are footing the bill.

George's metaphor for this process, for his parents wanting him to settle on a career path he hasn't chosen, is being put on a train, as we saw earlier in the chapter. The metaphor is apt, for a train moves along on rails with no divergence or detour or backtracking; it is on a set path. We find out later that George's father had also been put on a metaphorical train heading toward law school, the same train Mr. Richards's own father had been put on before him. Mr. Richards told George early on in the novel that he had known "as far back as fourth grade" that he wanted to go to law school, but we learn later that Mr. Richards's own father had pressured him into believing that. Mr. Richards seems to be a classic case of identity foreclosure. Aunt Sylvia reports that when her baby brother (George's future father) was brought home from the hospital, Grandpa Richards told her, "Here's your new brother, Sylvia, and someday he's going to be a partner in my firm" (*Gopher*, p. 183).

George's grandfather acknowledged his own identity foreclosure to George just before he had his stroke. The incident occurred late in the novel, after George had worked during his first year out of high school rather than going to college. " 'I've got to hand it to you, George,' he said. 'You always land on your feet.' He sat thinking for a minute, then added, 'There's something to be said for being your own man. Wish someone had said that to me when I was eighteen' " (*Gopher*, p. 168). Through several generations, this family has illustrated identity foreclosure. It took George's rebellious spirit and strength of character to break out of it.

Rather than succumb to his parents' pressure to get him on that train, George mixes one part stubbornness with two parts good judgment to take a year to sort out his conflicting thoughts about what he would like to do with his future—thus the "year of the gopher," George's version of a psychosocial moratorium. His decision to take this year off was formed at the time of his planned college visitation trip with his father to look over eastern private colleges. The trip itself was his father's decision, and the rules of engagement for the trip were also his father's, namely that his father would pick two schools to visit (Harvard and Yale), and George could pick one. He initially selected, jokingly, the University of Miami, but then settled on a prestigious private school he had heard of but knew nothing about, Swarthmore.

George intentionally rebels on this trip, messing up his interview at his father's alma mater, Harvard. "I felt miserable," George informs us, "but something told me that if I didn't stand up to him now, I'd be lost. If I let him put me on the old railroad, I'd never get off, and before you knew it, Jeri and Ollie would be on it, too" (*Gopher*, p. 43). His father had even helped, inadvertently, to show George how important it was to take some time for exploration. As he and Mrs. Richards emphasized the importance of his applications to Ivy League schools, he told George, "The thing you've got to remember is that you're going to be spending eight hours a day at a job for the rest of your life, so you'd better choose it carefully. All you do is figure out all the things you like to do—things you do best—put them together, and see what you come up with" (*Gopher*, p. 13).

Mr. Richards's formula sounds deceptively simple, but how does one go about figuring these things out? Obviously, one source of information about possible career options is through observation of parents. One of our students, whose father is a medical doctor and whose mother is a nurse practitioner, described his career search as a resolved commitment from early childhood to work in the medical field. While he may have explored many options during his education, this choice was always the most appealing.

Erikson (1968) observed that "in general it is the inability to settle on an occupational identity which most disturbs young people" (132). In this respect, George seems to be typical in his identity search. Mere observation of parental models probably does not qualify as genuine exploration of career options. During his moratorium year, his "year of the gopher," George provides readers with a number of clues about his thinking about occupational roles. He shows us his concern for his little brother, Ollie, and Ollie's likely learning disability. He objects vigorously when his parents force Ollie to sit at the kitchen table agonizing over his Spanish assignments. His objections lead to an argument with his father and to a final paternal outburst to get his own life in order before giving advice concerning Ollie. This outburst motivates George to fill out his college applications—albeit, we later learn, with a built-in self-destruct mechanism. When Ollie tells George that he wants to be a forest ranger, George seeks information that will be useful to Ollie in case he seriously wants to pursue that option.

Other clues to George's career exploration arise from his interaction with co-worker Shirl's daughter, Heather. Shirl, a divorcée who dotes on her daughter, also smothers her with unrealistic compliments and expectations. George sees clearly how Heather is not allowed to enjoy normal preadolescent friendships and pursuits. He subtly hints to both Shirl and Heather that he understands, saying to Heather at her birthday dinner, "And next year, when you're twelve, I hope your mom brings you back here again with a whole carload of friends, and you're the noisiest table in the room" (*Gopher*, p. 153). On another occasion, George takes Ollie to see a preadolescent gross-out movie, *The Revenge of the Termite People*. Shirl and Heather are also there, and Shirl engineers it so that Ollie and Heather sit together. Ollie and Heather are intensely embarrassed, and the outing is ruined for both of them. Shirl is oblivious to the situation, but George is acutely aware of it.

These are clues for the reader, but also for George. They are part of the exploration that this moratorium year illustrates for him. He describes his decision about a career path as a sudden revelation, but we know that it doesn't truly come out of nowhere because of the clues left along the way.

Thus, in the course of the novel, George goes from identity confusion to moratorium, and finally to identity achievement with respect to his occupational identity. Granted, he has a long way to go before he actually can function as a junior high school guidance counselor. But he seems sure that this direction is the right one for him, and the reader is convinced as well, even though it is possible George will ultimately change his mind. In an Eriksonian sense, it is not necessary to remain firmly fixed within a career direction, without any wavering, to be considered in the stage of identity achievement.

Influence of Earlier-Stage Resolutions

As we have said, resolutions of earlier normative crises leave their mark on personality. In adolescence, the outcome of the four previous normative crises will influence how this stage is experienced and how the crisis of identity will be resolved. We can therefore examine how George's functioning in adolescence betrays some elements of the first four normative crises that he has already experienced: trust vs. mistrust, autonomy vs. shame and doubt, initiative vs. guilt, and industry vs. inferiority.

Trust vs. Mistrust

The element of trust may influence the character of adolescence in a number of ways. In adolescence, one looks for heroes or role models in which to trust. Despite their pressure on him to adopt a life plan that he is skeptical about, George does love and admire his parents. He even takes in stride some of his father's belittling comments, such as "Four hundred million spermatozoa were racing for the ovum, and you're the one who got there first. Four hundred million other kids I could have had, and look what I got" (*Gopher*, p. 15).

That George does not trust his parents to make his life decisions for him is, ironically, a signal that they have been successful at parenting. George is right that they have been too focused on their own needs through the whole college-application debacle, and he tells them so. This scene forces George to become more independent, and to examine his own needs and values. His father essentially tells him he is on his own except for necessities, and George accepts the responsibility that goes with his newfound independence.

George's need for trust is played out more with his friends than with his parents. He is close enough to Dave ("Psycho") to share Dave's intimacies about his father's coming out, and he cares enough for him to try to fix him up with Maureen. Trust in ideals as well as people is an issue for identity. By the end of the novel, George has found an ideal—helping others through counseling—by which to prove himself trustworthy.

Autonomy vs. Shame and Doubt

The second stage ends with resolution of the crisis surrounding autonomy. In terms of identity, "the adolescent now looks for an opportunity to decide with free assent on one of the available or unavoidable avenues of duty and service, and at the same time is mortally afraid of being forced into activities in which he would feel exposed to ridicule or self-doubt" (Erikson, 1968, p. 129). The "free assent" phrase is important, and even essential to understanding George. George is exposed as having prepared his applications to the Ivy League colleges in such a way as to ensure his rejection. His parents ask why he didn't just tell them he didn't want to go to these colleges. George's answer shows the necessity of free assent to decisions about one's own identity: "I said it every way I knew how, but you weren't listening" (*Gopher*, p. 75).

On the other hand, George's stubborn decision not to go to the University of Minnesota (where he *was* accepted), just to spite his parents, shows his capacity for self-injury and his lack of mature, autonomous judgment. He is also highly susceptible to self-doubt. He cares enough about not going to college to mention that the school newspaper lists all the colleges his close friends will be attending but it puts the notation "work" beside his name. George also goes through a phase of intense self-doubt after the incident in which his friend Psycho almost drowns because George and others taunt him about his virginity. George becomes involved in the taunting because of his own feelings of inadequacy.

Initiative vs. Guilt

George shows considerable initiative in negotiating the stage of adolescence, as well as some guilt in his dealings with his peers. He finds a job as a helper at a garden center, the Green Thumb, and acquits himself well in the position. He leaves because Shirl, the older woman who works in the nursery office, comes on too strong in trying to initiate a sexual relationship with him. George gives notice to his boss, without explicitly turning Shirl in, and finds another job as a bicycle courier. He also does well at this job and boosts his self-image as an independent person by contributing some money to cover his "rent" at home.

But George also shows his capacity for guilt in the story. We have already described the guilt he expressed about his sexual relationship with Maureen. Although he wasn't "using" her any more than she was using him, he still felt guilty about having an intimate relationship with her for the sole purpose of gratifying his sexual impulses. His feelings of guilt were even more intense after the near-drowning incident with Psycho at the lake. After it was all over, and he was safely home in bed, he felt the real intensity of what could have been an immutable tragedy.

Industry vs. Inferiority

A favorable resolution of the normative crisis of the school years, industry vs. inferiority, is a sense of being able to do things well. George has opted for a career path in which he can make a difference, can do something well, and for him salary considerations are secondary. During the course of the novel, as George grows in maturity about his identity, his mother is reaching a new level of self-understanding as well. She has been working hard to get her master's degree. Now, she is reevaluating what that means to her, and she confides about it to George by telling him she plans to refuse an assignment for her degree because it would mean doing something she doesn't enjoy.

Mrs. Richards's situation indicates that one does not stop growing psychologically at some arbitrary age. One of the greatest strengths of Erikson's model is the notion that psychological growth is a life-cycle process and that what happens in later stages is influenced in significant ways by what has gone before.

Life Stage Issues in George's Family

Although our focus has been on George in our analysis of *The Year of the Gopher*, everybody in the family illustrates some important aspects of Erikson's life-cycle model. The story also shows how family dynamics affect individual personality trajectories. Remember that Erikson's theory is, first and foremost, an *interpersonal* theory. Thus, an analysis of some of the developmental dynamics of other family members is in order.

Mr. and Mrs. Richards

George's parents are in the generativity vs. stagnation stage in Erikson's life-cycle model. The primary concern of this stage is "establishing and guiding the next generation" (Erikson, 1968, p. 138). In a larger sense, the stage is about productivity and creativity in general. Both family and work provide a focus for this stage of life. George's parents are obviously very concerned about their children and their prospects in life. They have probably been too forceful in asserting their own wishes when guiding their children, so much so that George felt he had to rebel. He also felt bad about himself because he thought he was a disappointment to his parents.

And, as we have seen, George's mother has taken some important steps forward in her self-identity, reflected in her decision to emphasize generativity at work, through teaching, rather than salary and promotion. As the novel progresses, George's parents also learn that sometimes guiding the next generation must include knowing when to back off. When George quits his garden center job and takes on the bicycle courier job, he informs his parents of the basics of his decision without much detail, and they neither probe nor offer advice.

Trish, the Older Sister

Trish, the "Most Perfect Everything" in George's terminology, bridges the stages of identity vs. role confusion and intimacy vs. isolation. She is a student at Cornell who marries a summa cum laude graduate of Cornell after her second year. But despite her "perfection," she has an ulcer from the stress of trying to be perfect at everything. After her marriage, she works on her studies part time and works in a department store the rest of the time to support her husband through graduate school. The dilemma of combining career and family is a stronger one for women than men, and Trish seems to illustrate this dilemma even without yet having children. Erikson implied that there is a stronger link between identity and intimacy in women than in men.

Carol Gilligan is one of many theorists who regards Erikson's approach as attempting to define "woman's place in a man's life cycle," the title of one of her chapters in the book *In a Different Voice* (Gilligan, 1982). "Erikson's description of male identity as forged in relation to the world and of female identity as awakened in a relationship of intimacy with another person is hardly new," she says (Gilligan, 1982, p. 13). She goes on to say:

> Women's place in a man's life cycle has been that of nurturer, caretaker, and helpmate, the weaver of those networks of relationships on which she in turn relies. But while women have thus taken care of men, men have, in their theories of psychological development, as in their economic arrangements, tended to assume or devalue that care. (17)

Trish is a character whose experiences seem like those of many young women who must balance the expectations of family with their goals for their own independent achievement. She is a character with whom we empathize, and for whom we would like to suggest ways to restructure her life so that it could include less ulcer-causing stress.

Jeri, the Younger Sister

Jeri is also in high school, in Erikson's identity vs. role confusion stage. She is a straight-A student, with a reputation for being all-academic. Outside of school, she has begun testing limits and seems to be a little "wild." For example, George runs into her once at the 18–20 Club, a place where only people between the ages of 18 and 20 are admitted, supposedly. (George is just under 18 and Jeri is 16 at the time.) She is there with a guy George thinks to be about 20, with a Marine haircut. Jeri doesn't get home that night until after 2 A.M. Another night, George hears Jeri sneaking out of the house around 1 A.M.; she stays out all night.

By the end of the novel, we learn two things about Jeri. We learn that she hasn't really crossed the line too much in testing the limits. But the last incident recounted in the novel could have ended in disaster. She goes with a boy to his house when his parents are away, and he doesn't want to let her leave; he actually hits her hard enough to leave bruises. And, in a frank conversation between Jeri and George, we also learn that her limits testing has been a part of her own identity search. She is tired of being thought of as a "brain."

Some of Jeri's limits testing may illustrate Erikson's concept of "negative identity," which is "expressed in a scornful and snobbish hostility toward the roles offered as proper and desirable in one's family and environment" (Erikson, 1968, pp. 172–173). Being a brain has always been a model put forward as not just desirable, but almost necessary in the Richards family. Jeri wants to establish her uniqueness as an individual, something apart from the fairly narrow limits of acceptability in her family and school. Her decisions, therefore, are not necessarily well thought out, and she ultimately seems to reject the negative identity, at least in its strong and somewhat dangerous form.

Ollie, the Younger Brother

Ollie, at age 12, is near the end of the stage of industry vs. inferiority. Unfortunately, his resolutions to the dilemmas he has faced in this stage fall primarily within the inferiority outcome, at least early in the novel. His parents force him to take on academic assignments that he may not be suited for, such as Spanish. When he has difficulty with his assignments, his parents make him sit at the kitchen table and work until he completes them. During one such incident, George sees that Ollie is crying. When Ollie tells his mother he wants to drop Spanish, she labels that notion "ridiculous." " 'It's too *hard!*' Ollie said, a little louder, and I wondered if I was the only one who caught the quaver in his voice" (*Gopher*, p. 59).

After their grandfather's stroke, Ollie makes an observation, very uncharacteristic for a 12-year-old, that "life's short." George reminds him that their grandfather has had a good long life, living to age 73, and Ollie begins to muse about what that means to him. He figures that if he has to spend one-sixth of his life worrying about things like Spanish, he's only got half a life to do what he wants to do.

Ollie's struggle with a sense of inferiority are helped by a caring older brother, one who helps research requirements for forest ranger programs, which at that point in time is Ollie's major interest. However, because he has not yet even begun the crisis of identity, that interest may undergo modifications later. But George has given him the challenge, both as a role model who establishes a measure of independence and as a friend who challenges his assumptions. "Whose life is it, anyway?" George asks Ollie when Ollie demurs about being a forest ranger because of his father's potential disapproval.

Grandfather Richards

George's description of his grandfather at various family gatherings and holidays is of a rather crotchety and unpleasant person. At 73, widowed and retired, Grandpa Richards is in the last stage of the life cycle, ego integrity vs. despair. This stage is one of life review, and although he does not seem to be in despair, at the same time he appears to be somewhat short of full ego integrity. He is obviously engaged in a type of life review that is fairly depressive, muttering at Christmas about everyone eventually coming to dust. George tries to spend time with him, and in fact is watching football with him when Grandpa Richards has his stroke.

George's father and his aunt Sylvia argue over whether Grandpa Richards should move into a retirement home, with Mr. Richards taking the position that he should. The comparison to George's own life is not lost on him, as he listens in on the augment. Sylvia finally wins the argument. Basically, it's a quality-of-life argument, an argument over the essence of ego integrity. Sylvia convinces her brother that even if it's a mistake to let their father go back to his apartment, which is what he wants to do, we're all entitled to make mistakes.

SUMMARY

The crises and conflicts that the Richards family members experience seem "real" enough. They resonate with the experiences of people with whom we are familiar, and they serve as a case study in identity. George Richards is a young man who achieves a remarkable degree of psychological independence over the course of the events that constitute the novel *The Year of the Gopher*. He moves from identity confusion, to a psychosocial moratorium, and finally to commitments that qualify as identity achievement. Along the way, the rest of the family grows as well.

Among the other important messages of this novel is the notion that development occurs within a social system. The changes experienced by one family member influence other family members, for good or ill. In *The Year of the Gopher*, the changes are by and large positive ones for all members of the family.

By the end of this novel, George is on track for studying to be a guidance counselor, Ollie is excited about his prospects for becoming a forest ranger, Jeri sees how independence too early may come at too high a price, and Mrs. Richards discovers that her personal values are more important than monetary rewards. (We might wish for a better resolution for Trish, however.) All of these life changes can be understood within the framework of Erik Erikson's life-cycle approach to identity. Mr. Richards may have changed more than anyone else in the family. As the various individual normative crises settle into their respective resolutions, he tells his family that "the most marvelous thing about the human organism is its ability to change. . . . Maybe we've got enough lawyers in this family. There's something to be said for surprises, I guess" (*Gopher*, p. 200). The metaphorical train has by no means derailed, but the schedule and the destination are open for discussion.

RECOMMENDED READINGS

Fiction

Beake, Lesley. (1993). *Song of Be*. New York: Henry Holt. 94 pp. (ISBN: 0–8050–2905–2). MS.

There are so many ways in which Be feels caught. Is she a child or a young woman? Is she a Bushwoman, a follower of tribal ways, or a citizen of a Namibia struggling toward independence? When she heads into the desert to seek peace, Be is forced to find a way to balance ancient traditions with more modern ways of being in the world.

Bennet, James. (1994). *Dakota dream*. New York: Scholastic. 182 pp. (ISBN: 0–590–46680–1). HS.

In a dream, foster child Floyd Rayfield is told that he is really Charley Black Crow. As he pursues this vision, Floyd has to run from the authorities, who think he is dangerous, and from his past, in his attempt to figure out who he really is.

Castaneda, Omar S. (1994). *Imagining Isabel*. New York: Lodestar. 200 pp. (ISBN: 0–525–67431–4). HS.

Isabel knows that her dying mother wants her to marry Lucas. But the government of Guatemala wants the 16-year-old Mayan girl to leave her village and participate in a teacher-training program. As Isabel tries to balance her studies with caring for her younger sister, she must reconcile both her political world and her own desires.

Cooney, Caroline B. (1996). *The voice on the radio*. New York: Delacorte. 184 pp. (ISBN: 0–385–32213–5). MS.

Janie, who was kidnapped as a child in *The Face on the Milk Carton*, thinks her life is back on track. But the 16-year-old girl has to face a new challenge when her boyfriend, Reeve, uses his position as disc jockey for a college radio station to betray Janie and her family.

Danziger, Paula. (1980). *There's a bat in bunk five*. New York: Laurel Leaf. 150 pp. (ISBN: 0–440–98631–1). MS.

Marcy Lewis, of *The Cat Ate My Gymsuit*, is spending the summer as a camp counselor in training, for a group of talented young people. She's learning to deal with her new, more slender body and, in the process, is able to see that the father whom she has long hated has problems similar to her own.

Lynch, Chris. (1993). *Shadow boxer*. New York: HarperTrophy. 214 pp. (ISBN: 0–06–447112–8). MS.

When George was 9, his father, a professional boxer, died—killed by fighting. Now, at 14, George is concerned that his younger brother, Monty, seems to have boxing in his blood. What should George teach him about boxing, about love, and about how to be a man?

MacLachlan, Patricia. (1991). *Journey*. New York: Yearling. 83 pp. (ISBN: 0–440–40809–1). MS.

When Journey is 11, his mother runs away, leaving him and his sister with their grandparents. Using old photographs and a newly discovered skill as a photographer, Journey tries to put together a larger picture of his family's past.

Mazer, Norma Fox. (1997). *When she was good*. New York: Arthur Levine. 234 pp. (ISBN: 0–590–13506–6). HS.

When her horribly abusive and manipulative older sister dies, 17-year-old Em finds the courage to come to terms with her past, her parents, and her life with Pamela, her beloved sister.

Myers, Walter Dean. (1996). *Slam!* New York: Scholastic. 267 pp. (ISBN: 0–590–48667–5). HS.

At 17, "Slam" Harris thinks that, just maybe, his ability to slam-dunk may be his ticket into the world of pro sports. When Slam's coach confronts him with the realities involved in making it out of the inner city, Slam has to make some tough decisions about the kind of court on which he wants to play.

Nolan, Han. (1996). *Send me down a miracle*. New York: Harcourt Brace. 250. pp. (ISBN: 0–15–200978–7). MS.

Everyone expects Charity to follow in her father's footsteps and become a preacher. But then Charity meets Adrienne, who announces to the world that she has seen Jesus sitting in her house. Charity finds herself caught in the middle of the growing tensions between believers and nonbelievers, and questions almost every aspect of her life.

Nonfiction

Atkin, Beth. (1996). *Voices from the streets: Young former gang members tell their stories.* Boston: Little, Brown. 132 pp. (ISBN: 0–316–05634–0). MS.

Readers of these interviews with former gang members will develop a better appreciation for the ways a gang provides a sense of identity and security to young people.

Bode, Janet, and Stan Mack. (1994). *Heartbreak and roses: Real-life stories of troubled love.* New York: Delacorte. 158 pp. (ISBN: 0–385–32068–X). MS.

Readers of these interviews with teenagers begin to realize that a secure sense of self is a key ingredient in a successful relationship with someone else.

Cheney, Glenn Alan. (1995). *Teens with physical disabilities: Real-life stories of meeting the challenges.* Hillside, NJ: Enslow. 112 pp. (ISBN: 0–89490–625–9). MS.

Personal narratives provide glimpses into the lives of young people who have had to cope with almost every kind of physical problem.

Cole, Sheila. (1995). *What kind of love?: The diary of a pregnant teenager.* New York: Lothrup, Lee & Shepard. 192 pp. (ISBN: 0–688–12848–3). MS.

At 15, Val assumes she can have her baby and live an idyllic life with her boyfriend. But through her diary, she comes to terms with his abandonment and struggles to decide if her child would be better off in an adoptive home.

Gellman, Rabbi Marc, and Monsignor Thomas Hartman. (1995). *How do you spell God?: Answers to the big questions from around the world.* New York: Morrow. 206 pp. (ISBN: 0–688–13041–0). HS.

Trying to find answers to questions about religion and religious beliefs, TV's "God Squad" provides some strategies from around the world for dealing with such issues.

Hinojosa, Maria. (1995). *Crews: Gang members talk to Maria Hinojosa*. New York: Harcourt Brace. 168 pp. (ISBN: 0–15–292873). HS.

Hinojosa reports on her time spent hanging out with gang, or "crew" members, trying to find out why these young people are attracted to violence.

Landau, Elaine. (1994). *The beauty trap*. Riverside, NJ: Open Door/New Discovery/Silver Burdett. 128 pp. (ISBN: 0–02–751389–0). MS.

Landau explores the pressures young women face from the media and other elements of society to have perfect bodies and gorgeous faces.

Michelson, Maureen. (Ed.). (1994). *Women and work: In their own words*. New Sage. 191 pp. (ISBN: 0–939165–23–6). MS.

Women from all walks of life explore the ways in which their gender and their jobs have shaped their sense of self.

Nelson, Richard E., and Judith C. Galas. (1994). *The power to prevent suicide: A guide for teens helping teens*. Minneapolis: Free Spirit. 194 pp. (ISBN: 0–915793–70–9). HS.

Nelson and Galas provide lists of at-risk behaviors, discussion cues, questionnaires, and possible prevention techniques for adolescents concerned about their friends' mental health.

Tarpley, Natasha. (Ed.). (1995). *Testimony: Young African-Americans on self-discovery and black identity*. Boston: Beacon Press. 272 pp. (ISBN: 0–8070–0929–6). HS.

Essays, poems, and personal stories by young African Americans document the diversity of their experiences in coming to terms with their cultural heritage.

REFERENCES

Balistreri, E., N. A. Busch-Rossnagel, and K. F. Geisinger. (1995). Development and preliminary validation of the Ego Identity Process Questionnaire. *Journal of Adolescence* 18: 179–192.

Erikson, E. H. (1968). *Identity: Youth and crisis*. New York: Norton.

Gilligan, C. (1982). *In a different voice: Psychological theory and women's development*. Cambridge, MA: Harvard University Press.

Marcia, J. E. (1966). Development and validation of ego-identity status. *Journal of Personality and Social Psychology* 3: 551–558.

Marcia, J. E. (1983). Some directions for the investigation of ego development in early adolescence. *Journal of Early Adolescence* 3: 215–223.

Matthews, Steve. (1987). Review of *The Year of the Gopher*, by Phyllis Reynold Naylor. *School Library Journal* 33: 116.

Naylor, P. R. (1987). *The Year of the Gopher*. New York: Anthenum.

Rugow, A. M., J. E. Marcia, and B. R. Slugoski. (1983). The relative importance of identity status interview components. *Journal of Youth and Adolescence* 12: 387–400.

Schiedel, D. G., and J. E. Marcia. (1985). Ego identity, intimacy, sex role orientation, and gender. *Developmental Psychology* 21: 149–160.

Slugoski, B. R., J. E. Marcia, and R. F. Koopman. (1984). Cognitive and social interactional characteristics of ego identity statuses in college males. *Journal of Personality and Social Psychology* 47: 646–661.

CHAPTER 2

Identity through Body Image: Chris Crutcher's *Staying Fat for Sarah Byrnes*

Patricia L. Daniel and Vicki J. McEntire

INTRODUCTION

In our society, parents are credited with wanting their children to have better lives than they had. This is especially seen during adolescence, when most of today's adolescents are not having to work to contribute to the family's income. Many adolescents live in abundance: nice homes, designer clothes, cars, lots of friends, and well-stocked pantries and refrigerators. However, parents, teachers, businesspeople, doctors, lawyers, politicians, the military, advertisers, and the media contribute to sending a very unhealthy message to our adolescents: You must be thin to be loved, accepted, and successful. Furthermore, you must be free of any physical disfigurement in order to be considered for love, acceptance, and success. Your chances for success are higher if you are white, and your odds increase tremendously if you are male. Consequently, white males who were not born with cerebral palsy, epilepsy, multiple sclerosis, or other impairments, and who are not overweight have extremely high chances of being successful. White females who were born healthy and who are thin and attractive can also be successful.

What is the definition of "thin" or "attractive"? It is elusive, a moving target. The pictures of models in magazines portray extremely thin young people. What are the chances of average adolescents seeing someone who looks like themselves in one of these magazines? The message is clear when adolescents do not see themselves reflected in magazines, movies, and billboards: They are not good enough. So, they try to alter their appearance to look like the models portrayed. And as they try to alter their appearance, they have the applause and assistance of all the adults in their lives who want them to be successful, to look good.

Drawings in medical textbooks from the 1950s portray the naked female as rounder and heavier than do drawings from the 1990s. The changes in these drawings in medical textbooks may be a reflection of what females look like in the 1990s. Consider this: The Metropolitan Life Insurance Company published height and weight tables in 1959, and then revised and reissued tables in 1983. These tables were based on actuarial longevity figures compiled by the insurance industry. Ironically, the ideal weights were as much as eighteen pounds heavier for men and thirteen pounds heavier for women in the 1983 chart than they were in the 1959 chart (Matthews, 1991, pp. 7, 152–155). Therefore, at a time when we have research to indicate that being thin is unhealthy for a long life, we are sending the contradictory pictorial message that being thin is necessary for love, acceptance, and success.

Adolescence is a cultural phenomenon with its own subcultures of norms and values, dress codes, leisure activities, music, food, and language (Germain, 1991). It is most often the time of puberty, with rapid physiological changes, social crisis, and teens striving to be both "normal" and unique. These rapid changes lead to preoccupation with physical appearance.

SYNOPSIS

In *Staying Fat for Sarah Byrnes*, Chris Crutcher introduces us to 18-year-old Eric, who is terribly overweight, and his friend Sarah Byrnes, who at the age of 3 was severely burned on the face and hands when her father pushed her into a wood stove. Together, they struggle to understand themselves and how the world can be so cruel to both of them. Their trouble is compounded by the fact that Sarah, her face hideously scarred from her burning, sits alone and tormented in a hospital psychiatric ward. Eric, or "Moby" as he is known to his friends, finds time to loyally visit Sarah, until her psychotic father stalks Eric in an effort to learn his daughter's whereabouts. Learning of her father's attempts to find her, Sarah escapes, but not before her father stabs Eric. Eric recovers, brings her father to justice, and helps his friend Sarah find her way back into the world of love and acceptance.

A THERAPY SESSION WITH COACH LEMRY FROM
STAYING FAT FOR SARAH BYRNES

Often a third party can tell us more about individuals than the individuals themselves can. With this in mind, we have constructed what a therapy session might sound like between a therapist and Coach Lemry, a central figure in the lives of Eric and Sarah.

Therapist: I got your message about wanting to discuss what has happened with the Byrnes case. And by the way, congratulations on your new daughter! It sure sounds like Sarah could use a supportive family after what the media has said about her father.

Ms. Lemry: Thanks for seeing me on such short notice. Now that things have begun to settle, I wanted to talk to you and sort out how all of this happened. It has made a big impression on me to see how much pressure the school places on our students to give us a show of perfection, from academics to athletics. And, we don't even begin to prepare students to deal with their own or each other's physical imperfections or differences in thought.

Therapist: That's a complex issue, and certainly not one with easy answers. Let me make sure I understand. You're talking about how to prepare students to deal with how they perceive themselves and then to recognize how they influence what others think of themselves. Can you give me some examples?

Ms. Lemry: Sure, I can think of two clear examples from students I have had in class and on the swim team. In CAT class, Sarah challenged Mark Brittian to acknowledge that he preached the value of life but that he didn't display any value for her because of her scars, or for anyone else who thought differently from him. Mark resorted to his usual religious fortress but lost control when his former girlfriend, Jody, confronted him in class and told everyone how she had been pregnant with Mark's child and how Mark pushed her to have an abortion. When his own actions were exposed, he couldn't deal with others seeing his imperfections, and he attempted suicide by a drug overdose later that day.

Therapist: It sounds like Mark had to face himself and his imperfections in front of the class.

Ms. Lemry: Then there's "Moby," Eric Calhoun. He has been persecuted most of his life because of his weight, and now that he's lost weight from swimming, he is much more accepted by his peers. He and Sarah have been close friends. In junior high they were allies in waging the "war of the outcasts" (Crutcher, 1993, p. 31). Eric's dating someone now who years ago never noticed who he was.

Therapist: Wow! I'm surprised you haven't come to see me before now. Let's see if we can sort through some of this. It sounds as if the CAT class has been the catalyst for these kids to look beyond themselves. Tell me about it.

Ms. Lemry: CAT is a class in contemporary American thought offered as an elective to second-semester seniors who are willing to examine their beliefs, as Moby says it, "through a magnifying glass" (14). There are thirteen students in the class. I wanted to challenge the students to find the reasons for their own beliefs and to "put value back into words and ideas" (15). My role is to create a safe environment where any idea can be considered and to teach the students how to separate the ideas from the people who present them. I've told the students the class subtitle is "Accountability" (14) because they are accountable for everything they say.

Therapist: What an incredible class, and certainly needed, to challenge students to make their beliefs their own. The class is also small enough to allow everyone to participate. How difficult has it been to obtain and keep the administration's support?

Ms. Lemry: Funny you should ask that. The school principal, Mr. Patterson, has been supportive. It's Mautz, the vice-principal in charge of discipline, who seems to have the most difficulty with it. He attends the same church as Mark and Mark's family and views the religious arguments Mark makes as priority over the independent thinking of others. Mautz was sitting in on class the day Sarah and Jody confronted him. Mautz then came into class and attempted to imply CAT class and the members of the class were responsible for Mark's decision to attempt suicide. We didn't have time to process everyone's pain and reaction before the class was over. My main goal was to make sure the students knew they were not to blame for Mark's "responses to the world" (159).

Therapist: That's a lot to accomplish in a fifty-minute class period. Do you think you were successful in helping the students understand they were not to blame for Mark's suicide attempt? Do members of the class still blame themselves?

Ms. Lemry: I think many of them do know Mark is accountable for his own actions and that he made the choice to attempt suicide. Some of the students, especially the ones who share Mark's religious convictions and attend the same church, do think the class was too insensitive to Mark. I told the class Mark would need understanding when he returned to school and need to not be abandoned by them. But, their "guilt will only give him the mistaken belief that his actions were not of his own doing" (157).

Therapist: Good for you—and them. And all of this on top of the media coverage about Sarah's father and the abuse she endured, Mr. Byrnes and the assault and possible murder attempt of Eric, and the students' feelings about their responses to Sarah, Eric, and Mark. I'd certainly be willing to come to your class and help the students process what happened, but I think that would have been more effective if we had done that right after the events. What would be most helpful at this point is to give you some information and guidance on sorting through this, and you can pass that on to your students. You certainly have the rapport with them to be effective.

Ms. Lemry: That's why I'm here to talk to you. I can teach the students and challenge them to think independently. The class is set up to teach the students to examine their beliefs and to realize the power of their words. I want to take this a step further and talk about how we decide what we think of ourselves and how our words and actions impact other people.

Therapist: As I said, that's a very complex issue. Especially if you are trying to accomplish that in a class of adolescents whose egos are developmentally at a fragile time. The other critical piece is that one's self-image begins forming early in life, from infancy onward. The most influential people are the family, the caregivers. Some caregivers are nurturing, encouraging, and can lead children a long way to feeling good about themselves. Others foster negative self-images by the nature of how the family is structured, and by how much support and nurturing a child receives from immediate family, extended family, and even the community. It's a difficult task to take an adolescent, or even an adult, who hasn't grown up in an accepting, nurturing environment and then teach the person how to have a positive self-image.

Ms. Lemry: I know this seems more important to me now because Sarah has joined our family. She's had such a difficult childhood, without even mentioning the disfiguring scars on her face and hands.

Therapist: Tell me about Sarah. The media coverage was brief and hor-rific.

Ms. Lemry: Sarah is an only child. She lived with her mother and father until she was 3; that's when her father intentionally burned her. Sarah has good memories of her mother dressing her up, taking her to the park, reading stories to her. She also remembers special times when she and her mother would comfort each other after her father had beaten her mother. From what Sarah has said, her mother and father had really violent fights, hitting and throwing things. One particular night, Sarah's mother fought back and was threatening to kill Sarah's father. Her father had her mother by the hair and had filled the kitchen sink with water. Sarah was hiding under the stairs, watching her father continually dunk-ing her mother's head in the sink. Sarah was afraid he would kill her mother and she would be left alone with him. She ran from under the stairs and crashed into his legs. He loosened the grip on her mother. She got away, got a knife from the drawer, and came after him. Mr. Byrnes held Sarah in front of him and backed down the hallway into the living room. Sarah remembers him saying, "Here's your pretty little baby for you" (104), and then he put her face into the hot stove. I'm sure her hands went up in reflex. The next thing Sarah remembers is waking up in the hospital. Her father said she had pulled a pot of spaghetti off the stove onto herself.

Therapist: Were the child protective authorities called?

Ms. Lemry: Sarah remembers them asking questions about his story and the inconsistency with the injuries. She was too afraid to tell them what happened because Mr. Byrnes told Sarah her mother was gone and would never be back. He also told her if she told what happened, he'd burn the rest of her. He didn't care what they did to him. The bastard even refused to allow the doctors to do any reconstructive surgery unless it was med-ically necessary.

Therapist: It's so hard to imagine anyone intentionally hurting their child. What about Sarah's mother. Did he kill her?

Ms. Lemry: Sarah thought for a while she was dead, but then decided her father wouldn't be so stupid as to do that. The police were already asking questions, and if her mother couldn't be found, it would make him look more responsible for her injuries. She thinks her father burned her face so her mother wouldn't want her anymore. No more pretty baby. Some of Sarah's other memories of her father's parenting skills were that he'd tie her up and withhold food from her. God, I hate him for all the things he put her through!

Therapist: I can understand why you would hate him. So Sarah's father was not only cruel to her directly, but the physical scars also brought emotional scars, kids teasing her, and Sarah not fitting in with her peers.

Ms. Lemry: Sarah didn't fit in with anyone but Eric. He was overweight and she had a scarred, disfigured face. She says they both shared the "terminal uglies" (17). When they were in junior high, Sarah made everyone call her Sarah Byrnes because she hated waiting for "every new Einstein at school thinking he was the only genius in the world to figure out this great pun about her last name and her condition" (7).

Therapist: It doesn't sound like Sarah got what she needed from her father, or absent mother, to develop a positive self-image, especially a positive body image. Tell me about Eric and his friendship with Sarah.

Ms. Lemry: Eric's nickname has been "Moby" for years, even now that he's lost weight. He was overweight until about a year after he started swimming on the team. Eric and Sarah had been good friends, social outcasts together for a long time. They waged war the only way they could against those who tormented them. They put together an underground newspaper in the eighth grade to get back at another student who had beaten Sarah up trying to get her lunch money. They called the thing *Crispy Pork Rinds*, saying Sarah was crispy, Eric was a porker, and the rinds were the things left over that nobody wanted. There were other tactical assaults on those they felt wronged by: "a box of fish guts planted in a locker here at the beginning of a long weekend, analgesic balm spread lavishly there in someone's underpants while he was dressed down for PE" (67), and hollow gumballs filled with Tabasco sauce with a hypodermic syringe.

Therapist: They certainly sound creative!

Ms. Lemry: Sarah was afraid Eric would go away when he lost weight. She told him, "People will just look at you differently than they do now. Other people will like you, and you'll go to them" (68). I couldn't figure out how Eric was swimming four to six thousand yards a day and still not losing weight. He later told me he had been staying fat for Sarah Byrnes. For Sarah, Eric's losing weight would mean he would "get svelte and handsome and popular" (67) and she'd have to hate him. Eric didn't want to lose Sarah's friendship.

Therapist: But from what I've heard and read, Eric didn't go away from Sarah after he lost weight.

Ms. Lemry: No. He never did. They did spend less time together because of Eric's swimming schedule for meets and practices. But Eric was determined to prove to Sarah he was committed to their friendship. He says he still stays fat for Sarah by refusing any invitations that exclude her, and he doesn't associate with anyone who isn't willing to include her.

Therapist: Have there been any other people for Sarah who have accepted her for who she is and not judged her on her physical appearance?

Ms. Lemry: Sarah's intelligent, and I know she got some positive feedback from teachers throughout school. She's developed a quick and sometimes biting wit to deal with others. But she's been left out of so much social interaction with her peers because of her scars. We've talked at home about how the things others say about us affect how we feel about ourselves. Sarah brought up another perspective with Mark and Mautz, that sometimes it's what others don't say to us that sends a clear message we are not okay. She told Mark she could count "on an amputee's fingers" (151) the number of times he'd spoken to her and said Mautz had never said anything to her, in spite of Sarah's being an honor student. She really nailed them both for talking about how sacred life is and not acknowledging her own life.

Therapist: I think you and Sarah are on the right track. As children and adults, a significant amount of how we look at ourselves is determined by the perspectives of the people we are around. These social messages are then integrated into our own self-messages. There are three results: the self we once were; the self we can and cannot become; and the self we and others see at the moment. For Sarah, there is the self she once was; Sarah without the scars. That Sarah was loved and nurtured by her mother.

Ms. Lemry: She remembers the feelings from her mother she thinks is love. Sarah also says everyone told her and her mother she was really pretty.

Therapist: Then there's the Sarah with the scars, the Sarah she and her peers see her being at the moment. That Sarah has focused most of her life on having the "terminal uglies" (17). Children can be cruel, or brutally honest, in what they say and how they act. Adults can also be cruel, most often in a less honest way, like Mautz never speaking to Sarah. The key is to understand the cyclical pattern of behavior and response. It sounds like Sarah's only positive images of herself to draw upon came from some of her teachers and from Eric, another social outcast. Since Sarah has such limited positive images to draw on, the negative image is going to be the pervasive, strongest one. It's a basic instinct to protect herself, even if she views the self she's protecting as negative. Sarah then projects that negative image into the future. She anticipates, seeks, and elicits negative perspectives from others. When she gets what she expects, it reinforces the negative view and thoughts she has about herself. Sarah focuses on what she cannot become, and she cannot see what she can become. Then the entire cycle starts again.

Ms. Lemry: So how does it ever stop? Even if the doctors can do any reconstructive or plastic surgery now, Sarah will never physically be beautiful again and will still have the internal scars after any of the others heal. How can she ever shift her focus to what she can become and develop a positive self-image?

Therapist: It won't be easy, yet it's not impossible for Sarah to have a positive self-image. Think of the obstacles we have to overcome in order to develop a positive self-image. There's the media blitz we get every day. Only the "pretty" people are chosen to model clothing and other products in magazines. Only the "pretty" people are seen in the leading, hero or heroine, roles on television. The "ugly" people are most often the villains, the poor, the outcasts.

Ms. Lemry: You're right. I can't think of a movie I've seen where the good guys were disfigured or even overweight.

Therapist: Think about product marketing along with that. For an overweight person, or even a larger person who is taller than the norm, clothing can't be purchased in most department stores. Some larger department store chains have responded by adding a specialty area within the store where other-sized clothing may be purchased. Typically, the selection is small, and the colors and prints are drab. That continues to reinforce the image that other-sized people shouldn't or don't want to be noticed.

Ms. Lemry: That's especially difficult for adolescents, with the pressure, and expense, of wearing the "right" designer clothes. Tommy Hilfiger and Polo don't come in plus sizes except in men's shirts and slacks. Some of the designer clothing is cut small, some is more generous.

Therapist: The issue about developing a positive body image goes well beyond your classroom, Cindy. We talked about how we decide what we think of ourselves. I would recommend individual therapy for Sarah, and some young adult literature portraying teens with physical differences in a positive light, to help speed the process of her developing a positive body image and self-image. Family therapy could also be beneficial in helping you, your husband, and Sarah communicate your feelings and adjust to the changes of your family structure. I can't give you any clear-cut answers to the second part of your question: how to increase the students' awareness of how their words and actions impact people. I do think you are giving your students an excellent start by challenging them to put words to their beliefs. We also need to challenge the media through our communities to portray realistic people in realistic roles.

INTERVENTIONS

Adults in our society need to lead the way in helping adolescents develop healthy body images, by consciously portraying the rich diversity encompassed by a healthy body image. One can have a healthy body image and have (or be):

- dark brown skin
- light brown skin
- yellow skin
- white skin
- curly hair
- straight hair
- full lips
- thin lips
- slanted eyes
- almond-shaped eyes
- a small nose
- a large nose
- a round nose
- a pointed nose
- a tall frame
- a short frame
- heavy

- skinny
- a physical impairment including, for example:
    - polio
    - cerebral palsy
    - epilepsy
    - diabetes
    - scoliosis
- gay
- straight

The adults in our society need to challenge the media to portray realistic people in realistic roles. We need to look critically at the propaganda that we have been fed for years and demand a healthier diet!

There are many books and resources that address body image in general, and then many more books that address specific aspects of body image. We want all young people to be able to see themselves in literature so that they know they are not alone. Literature reinforces how we think about ourselves.

RECOMMENDED READINGS

Fiction

Blume, Judy. (1973). *Deenie*. New York: Laurel Leaf. 144 pp. (ISBN: 0–440–93259–9). MS, HS.

At 13, Deenie is diagnosed with scoliosis and must wear a brace for four years to prevent her from being permanently handicapped. Deenie's dad is a source of strength, and she discovers that she is stronger than she had realized.

Blume, Judy. (1974). *Blubber*. New York: Dell. 153 pp. (ISBN: 0–440–90707–1). ES, MS.

Jill and her well-to-do friends nickname Linda "Blubber" because she is overweight. Jill feels powerful as Blubber performs humiliating tasks: kissing Wendy's sneakers and lifting up her skirt. Suddenly, however, Jill is alienated by her friends and is attacked with glee.

Crutcher, Chris. (1987). *The Crazy Horse Electric Game*. New York: Greenwillow. 215 pp. (ISBN: 0–688–06683–6). MS, HS.

Willie Weaver must learn to live in his handicapped body after a boating accident ends his athletic career. He is impatient with himself and feels like a burden to his parents and an embarrassment to his girlfriend. In time, though, Willie learns much about himself, his strength, and how to cope.

Danziger, Paula. (1988). *The Cat Ate My Gymsuit*. New York: Laurel Leaf. 119 pp. (ISBN: 0–440–91612–7). ES, MS.

Marcy Lewis is a shy, overweight 13-year-old. She does not have friends at school, and she expends much energy thinking of reasons why she cannot dress out in PE class. The new English teacher, Ms. Finney, helps Marcy recognize her worth as an individual.

Feuer, Elizabeth. (1990). *Paper Doll*. New York: Farrar, Straus & Giroux. 185 pp. (ISBN: 0–374–35736–6). MS, HS.

After losing her legs in a car accident ten years prior, Leslie Marx has played the violin. Music becomes drudgery until she meets Jeffrey, a student with cerebral palsy, who encourages her to play. Leslie discovers that her love for music is real and that giving and receiving love are real also.

Greene, Constance C. (1986). *Just Plain Al*. New York: Viking Kestrel. 134 pp. (ISBN: 0–670–81250–1). MS, HS.

Al(exandra) frets over turning 14 and being plain and physically undeveloped. She wants to change her name so she will appear more sophisticated. By the end of the book, Al has accepted that her name has little to do with who she is and that what is important is that she do the best she can do.

Greene, Constance C. (1988). *Monday I Love You*. New York: Harper & Row. 170 pp. (ISBN: 0–06–022183–6). MS, HS.

Grace Schmitt is a 15-year-old who wears a size 38-D bra. Her classmates tease her and play pranks on her. To escape their torment, Grace daydreams of being rich and living a life of pleasure. Throughout the book are memories of her childhood that provide the reader with insights into her low self-esteem and why she endures her classmates' cruelty.

Levenkron, Steven. (1991). *The Best Little Girl in the World.* New York: Warner. 253 pp. (ISBN: 0–446–35865–7). MS, HS.

Kessa is a 15-year-old who suffers from anorexia nervosa. She keeps all the pictures of the thinnest models from magazines and says to them, "Soon I'll be thinner than all of you. The thinner is the winner." Kessa almost completely stops eating because she believes her five-foot-four-inch, ninety-eight-pound body is ugly and overweight.

Lipsyte, Robert. (1977). *One Fat Summer.* New York: HarperKeypoint. 232 pp. (ISBN: 0–06–447073–3). MS, HS.

Bobby Marks is an overweight 14-year-old who has made an art of hiding his body by wearing baggy clothes and swimming underwater when his parents force him to go to the lake. His best friend, Joanie, goes to New York City to have her nose operated on. Bobby gets a job cutting the lawn on a large estate. The job taxes his physical strength and eventually helps him develop a strong sense of who he is.

Stren, Patti. (1986). *I Was 15-Year-Old Blimp.* New York: Signet. 160 pp. (ISBN: 0–451–14577–1). MS, HS.

Gabby decides she must lose weight in order to secure a particular boy's attention. She begins taking laxatives and purging her meals. When her parents become aware, they send her to a camp for people with eating disorders. Readers become acquainted with some of the help that is available for people who have bulimia.

Nonfiction

Abraham, Suzanne, and Derek Llewellyn-Jones. (1992). *Eating Disorders: The Facts*, 3rd ed. New York: Oxford University Press. 201 pp. (ISBN: 0–19–262199–8). MS, HS.

The authors, gynecologist/obstetricians who also work with patients in an eating disorders unit, write concisely about anorexia nervosa, bulimia nervosa, and obesity. Case histories are provided, as well as excerpts from patients' journals and letters.

Boston Women's Health Book Collective. (1992). *The New Our Bodies. Ourselves: A Book by and for Women*. New York: Simon & Schuster. 752 pp. (ISBN: 0–671–79176–1). HS.

The first chapter is titled "Body Image." It exposes American culture's preoccupation with telling women and girls how they *should* look.

Brown, Catrina, and Karin Jasper. (Eds.). (1993). *Consuming Passions: Feminist Approaches to Weight Preoccupation and Eating Disorders*. Toronto: Second Story. 459 pp. (ISBN: 0–929005–42–2). HS, A.

This collection of essays written by therapists, community workers, and activists promotes ways to practice a fat-positive, nondiscriminatory, and pro-woman approach to life.

Emme, Daniel Paisner. (1996). *True Beauty: Positive Attitude and Practical Tips from the World's Leading Plus-Size Model*. New York: Putnam. 259 pp. (ISBN: 0–399–14204–5). HS, A.

Emme speaks to the reader about how she accepted her body, which is larger than that of the models portrayed as the ideal size, and then speaks as an ambassador for all people who do not fit into the small, narrow box that is proclaimed as the ideal.

Freedman, Rita. (1988). *Bodylove: Learning to Like Our Looks—and Ourselves*. New York: Harper & Row. 256 pp. (ISBN: 0–06–016025–X). MS, HS.

This is a straightforward, easy-to-read book that takes into account the many aspects of body image: visual, mental, emotional, kinesthetic, historical, and social.

Hillman, Carolynn. (1996). *Love Your Looks: How to Stop Criticizing and Start Appreciating Your Appearance*. New York: Simon & Schuster. 303 pp. (ISBN: 0–684–81138–3). HS.

The author presents a concise but scathing account of how corporate America, the media, and family and friends have portrayed women as all the same size and their beauty as one-dimensional.

Johnson, Julie Tallard. (1991). *Celebrate You!: Building Your Self-Esteem*. Minneapolis: Lerner. 72 pp. (ISBN: 0–8225–0046–9). MS, HS.

The author writes that self-esteem includes our thoughts, feelings, beliefs, and desires, and she proclaims that positive self-esteem is a deep acceptance of self, despite shortcomings, mistakes, or disabilities. There is a self-esteem quiz with an explanation of what a score above a certain number might indicate.

Kaufman, Gershen, and Lev Raphael. (1990). *Stick Up for Yourself!: Every Kid's Guide to Personal Power and Positive Self-Esteem*. Minneapolis: Free Spirit. 81 pp. (ISBN: 0–915793–17–2). MS, HS.

The majority of this short book deals with getting and using personal power. The four parts of personal power presented are: (1) being responsible (for one's own behavior and one's own feelings), (2) making choices, (3) getting to know oneself, (4) getting and using power in relationships and life.

Lemberg, Raymond. (Ed.). (1992). *Controlling Eating Disorders with Facts, Advice, and Resources*. Phoenix, AZ: Oryx. 218 pp. (ISBN: 0–89774–691–0). MS, HS, A.

Acknowledging the societal pressures to look slim and trim, the authors identify causes, symptoms, and effects of eating disorders.

LeShan, Eda. (1992). *What Makes You So Special?* New York: Dial Books for Young Readers. 145 pp. (ISBN: 0–8037–1155–7). MS, HS.

This book addresses the effect of heredity as well as that of the nurture of family, friends, and teachers. The author relates stories of her life, including family members, teachers, and friends.

Levine, Saul, and Kathleen Wilcox. (1986). *Dear Doctor*. New York: Lothrop, Lee & Shepard. 265 pp. (ISBN: 0–688–07095–7). MS, HS.

This book is organized into chapters made up of letters young people wrote to "Youth Clinic," a nationally syndicated column. The two doctors offer sensitive, sensible answers to teenagers' most troubling questions about a wide variety of issues.

REFERENCES

Crutcher, C. (1993). *Staying Fat for Sarah Byrnes*. New York: Greenwillow.

Germain, C. B. (1991). *Human Behavior in the Social Environment: An Ecological View*. New York: Columbia University Press.

Granvold, D. K. (Ed.). (1994). *Cognitive and Behavioral Treatment: Methods and Applications*. Pacific Grove, CA: Brooks/Cole.

Matthews, J. R. (1991). *Library in a Book: Eating Disorders*. New York: Facts On File.

CHAPTER 3

Sexual Identity: M. E. Kerr's *Deliver Us from Evie*

Rita G. Drapkin and Lynne B. Alvine

INTRODUCTION

> The seniors are out to get you. They call "SOU-weeee! Pig, pig, pig!" at you, and they put you in a trash can, tie the lid with a rope, and kick you around in it. . . . That happened to me first thing in the morning. I was a transfer junior from Duffton. Then, in the afternoon, a few got me by my locker. They read my name on the door, PARR BURRMAN, and one of them said, "Hey, we know your brother. What's his name again?"
>
> "Doug Burman," I said.
>
> They said, "Not *that* brother! Your other brother."
>
> "I only have one brother," I said.
>
> They said, "What about Evie?"
>
> Then they began to laugh. They began to say things like "You remember *him*, don't you? Doesn't he live with you? Sure he does! The Burrman brothers: Doug, Parr, and Evie!" (Kerr, 1994, 1)

For most teenagers, nothing could be worse than not "fitting in" with the group. Perhaps the inherent conflict of trying to discover one's identity and still be like others creates turmoil for many adolescents. Depending on the individual, conforming to family or societal standards may be more or less difficult. The families and communities in which adolescents live may vary in their levels of openness toward differences. With many aspects of teenage life, there is often a broad range of what is acceptable. Not so with sexual identity.

In the United States, as in most of the world today, heterosexuality is the norm. Young people who are not heterosexual are often considered different, weird, abnormal, strange. They are frequently the targets of school bullies or the victims of hate crimes. Teenagers often hurl the term "faggot" as a put-down, often without any conscious regard for the other individual's sexual identity. For some adolescents, the label is simply another verbal weapon available to be used in a moment of defense or anger. A Harris Poll, released in 1992, revealed that 86% of high school students would be very upset if classmates called them gay or lesbian.

Sometimes such terms are used against those who fit the stereotype of a gay male or lesbian; sometimes they are directed toward—or overheard by—those struggling with their sexual identity. Because most gay, lesbian, and bisexual young people grow up in social contexts steeped in homophobic prejudice, they often internalize antigay beliefs. The result is often the development of low self-esteem or even self-hatred. An additional complication is the isolation experienced by gay, lesbian, and bisexual people, particularly teens and young adults. Gay youths fear that coming out to others will result in rejection. According to documentation by the Department of Health and Human Services (*60 Minutes*, March 1, 1998), one out of four gay and lesbian teens who disclose their sexual orientation to their families are thrown out of their homes.

Unlike racial and ethnic minority individuals who are born into families like themselves, sexual minority youth often feel different from others in their own homes, as well as from people at school and others in their community. It is not unusual for a gay person to spend most or all of the teen years without ever having met another identifiable gay or lesbian person. Sexual minority youth rarely see themselves reflected in what they read or view on television or in movies. Thus, appropriate adult role models—happy, healthy, fully actualized gay men and lesbians—are lacking for these youths.

Self-hatred and isolation can be a deadly combination. A number of studies have shown that the rate of suicide among gay, lesbian, and bisexual teens is significantly higher than that of heterosexual teens. As noted in the *Report of the Secretary's Task Force on Youth Suicide*, released by the Department of Health and Human Services in 1989, gay and lesbian youth are two to three times more likely to commit suicide than heterosexual youth (Remafedi, 1994).

Fortunately, there have been major changes in the past two decades. In 1997, approximately 36 million people witnessed Ellen DeGeneres's coming out as a lesbian in her role as the star of *Ellen*, a prime-time sitcom, and in her personal life. More and more corporations and municipalities are providing benefits to partners of gay and lesbian employees. It is expected that Hawaii will soon grant gays and lesbians the right to marry. But such hard-won gains toward equal rights are inevitably met by a conservative backlash. The Baptist Church organized a boycott against Disney for its provision of partner benefits as well as its sponsorship of the television show *Ellen*. At the beginning of 1998, laws that prevent legal recognition of the marriages of those couples who fly to Hawaii to tie the knot had been passed in twenty-seven states. The progressive social shifts that have come about have occurred unevenly across the country. They may be unknown and unrealized by a teen growing up in middle America. Most kids struggling with their sexual identity still do so under a cloak of silence and shame.

Deliver Us from Evie touches upon many of these issues. It does so with little threat to the young adult reader, who may find the topic of sexual identity frightening. For the teacher who wishes to introduce the topic of sexual orientation to students without alarming administrators or parents, this novel offers minimal risk. *Deliver Us from Evie* includes no explicit sexual scenes. It also may be "safer" for classroom use because of Kerr's use of point of view. The protagonist, Parr Burrman, is a 15-year-old, white, heterosexual high school freshman—a "normal" kid, a member of the dominant culture. It is through his eyes that readers are invited to consider the themes of identity, stereotypes, love, and betrayal.

SYNOPSIS

The Burrmans are like many families in Duffton, Missouri. They own a farm; their kids go to school during the day and work on the farm after school and on the weekends. They worry about paying off their mortgage, and they try to stay on the good side of Mr. Duff, the local banker for whose family the town is named. There are three Burrman children: Parr, Evie, and Doug, who are 15, 18, and 20, respectively. Parr is a high school freshman, Evie has graduated from high school and works on the farm full time, and Doug is attending the agricultural college at the University of Missouri. Initially, we learn that Parr is the only one of the three children who does not want to be a farmer. Throughout the story, he struggles with his sense of identity, which appears to be in conflict with what he believes to be family and community expectations for him. Evie loves farming and can repair anything. She is preparing to go to the agricultural college, like Doug, to learn all she can about working on the land. Evie is good-natured and is quick to do favors for others, like offering to give Parr rides before he has a driver's license. Evie seems to get along well with everyone, especially with her dad. They work side by side, constantly trading jokes. Evie's appearance, however, is a source of constant irritation to her mother. Mrs. Burrman's concerns stem mostly from her stereotype of gay and lesbian people, and her desire for her daughter to live a happy, "normal" life.

Cord Whittle is a young man who works for the Burrmans, helping them with harvesting and planting. He is attracted to Evie, whose mother is always trying to fix them up. Patsy Duff, the attractive 17-year-old daughter of the local banker, also pursues Evie. When Mr. Duff learns that his daughter is spending time with Evie, he becomes angry and tells Evie to stay away from Patsy. Parr and his mother have a frank discussion about the situation.

"Does Mr. Duff think Evie's a dyke?"

"I hate that word, Parr. . . . Someone like Evie gets the blame when there's suspicion of such a thing."

"Do *you* think she's one?"

"That's crossed my mind, Parr. You've heard me nagging at her about trying to be more of a lady. Of course it's crossed my mind."

"What if she is one?"

"It's going to be very hard for her if she is."

"It'll be hard for both of them, won't it?"

"It'll be harder for Evie. Evie can't pass herself off as something else. It isn't in her nature." (65)

Doug falls in love with a sorority girl who does not want to be a farmer's wife, so he changes his major to veterinary medicine. Parr becomes attracted to Angel, a young girl whose family worships at a different church; they begin to date. Despite threats from Mr. Duff, Patsy and Evie continue to see each other secretly. Evie confides in Parr about the relationship. Parr continues to defend Evie to others and tries to encourage his mother to get off Evie's case. Among other things, Evie shares with Parr her dawning realization that she will not be able to be herself and live happily in Duffton. With Doug deciding not to be a farmer and Evie thinking about leaving, Parr begins to feel trapped.

Parr begins to blame Patsy for what he sees as his inevitable future as a farmer. With the help of a few beers, Cord conspires with Parr to

make Evie and Patsy's relationship much more public. The result they
are hoping for is that Mr. Duff will send Patsy away, that Evie will
forget all about Patsy and go back to farming, and, most important, that
Cord's and Parr's lives will return to normal. Together, Cord and Parr
put a sign on the veteran's memorial in the center of town that says
"Evie loves Patsy and vice versa." As they predict, the whole town now
knows about the relationship and "old man Duff," who is enraged, plans
to send Patsy off to Europe. What they don't plan for is that the sheriff
will tell Evie to stop seeing Patsy, that Evie will flee Duffton, that Parr's
parents will realize Cord's role in the "prank," and that Angel's family
will become concerned about Evie's influence on Angel. Most of all,
Parr does not anticipate how guilty and ashamed he will feel for having
betrayed his sister. In the end, Patsy runs away to join Evie in New York
City and, as the novel ends, they are both trying to mend fences with
their respective families.

INTERVENTION

For a variety of reasons, it is unlikely that any of the characters in
this novel would present themselves for traditional intervention with a
mental health practitioner. The small town of Duffton is drawn as relatively unsophisticated and homogeneous. Despite major advances over
the last couple of decades, a stigma remains on the related mental health
fields of psychiatry, psychology, and social work in our culture, especially in small towns such as Duffton. If guidance were sought from any
professional, it would most likely be either from a member of the clergy,
a family physician, or a teacher. Ministers, doctors, and teachers who
left town for their graduate work may have developed broader views.
They were, however, raised in the same town, and some may still hold
similar values as the majority of the community and/or they may not
have overcome their own internalized homophobia. Influenced by personal or religious beliefs, and lacking appropriate training, many professionals may offer a discouraging picture to individuals who are
struggling with sexual orientation. Studies (Coleman, 1982; Harbeck,
1992) show that many gay, lesbian, and bisexual individuals have been
offered a range of damaging "help," including violation of their confi-
dences; provision of information to family members; condemnation for
same-gender sexual behavior; and offers of "cures" via conversion therapy or exorcism. If assistance were sought from a mental health practitioner in a town such as Duffton, the most likely scenario would be that

either one or both sets of parents (the Burrmans and the Duffs) would pressure their daughters into seeking help for their "problem."

Given what we believe is the status quo in small towns such as Duffton with regard to attitudes toward mental health treatment, we want to suggest options that are more accessible and more realistic for the characters of this novel in the community context in which they live. First we will consider intervention, that is, what might be helpful once events such as those in the story have already unfolded. After this, we will consider prevention, or what conditions in an environment such as Duffton might have brought about a different outcome for the story.

Parr

Parr is dealing with a number of identity struggles in the novel, all of which would be considered developmentally appropriate. According to Erikson (1963), it is during adolescence that answering the question "Who am I?" becomes crucial. The process of individuation includes developing one's own values and seeing oneself as an individual apart from one's family and peers. Most adolescents, in order to individuate from their families, need a reference or peer group with whom they can identify. When adolescents feel very different from their peers and do not have a sense of belonging, they lack a sense of social identity. This void can often interfere with, or delay, other developmental tasks necessary to help them move forward with life.

The Burrman children have been raised in a family business, farming. Accordingly, Parr feels pressured to consider the good of the whole (his family) over the good of the individual (himself). For Parr, the struggle is especially difficult because he is a considerate person and tends to be a people pleaser. As presented in the novel, Parr's family loyalty overrides his need to identify with his peers. Perhaps if Parr had been confused about his own sexuality, or if he were more peer identified than family identified, he would have been less accepting of his sister. It is only when Evie's sexuality impacts directly on Parr's own identity struggle that he acts against her.

Parr's life is affected by Evie's sexual orientation in at least three arenas: he is harassed at school; he is afraid he will be trapped in a life of being a farmer; and his girlfriend's family, based on their religious beliefs, are concerned about Evie's influence. Parr's decision to make Evie's relationship public is influenced by alcohol and by Cord, a man with his own agenda—his attraction to Evie. The combination of these factors is more than Parr, at the age of 15, can handle on his own. Parr's actions bring him shame because they go against what he knows, in his own heart, are his own values of family loyalty and respect for others. The novel does not even deal with the possible consequences of Parr's role in the incident bring uncovered, had they been.

What were Parr's options for finding support as he tried to understand his sister's situation and its impact on him? One problem was that Parr did not know anyone else who was gay or lesbian other than Joe, a cousin on his father's side. Parr had heard his father refer to him as "Cousin Josephine" and knew his father thought of Uncle Joe and his male companion as a "couple of fruits." Like most kids, Parr was attuned to his parents' values, and most likely these clues deterred any discussion with his father. Parr also knew that Mrs. Burrman was uncomfortable with Evie's nontraditional behavior. Parr was irritated by his mother's attempts to change Evie, and, as Evie's only confidant in the family, he probably would have felt disloyal in sharing Evie's secrets with his mother. Most adolescents are uncomfortable discussing sexuality with adults, especially their parents. Thus, as is typically the case with young people, Parr chose not to share his very personal questions with his parents. Parr did not seem to know anyone who had a relative or friend whom they knew to be gay or lesbian. So despite the fact that Parr was not, himself, a member of a sexual minority group, he was still isolated when it came to dealing with his feelings about his sister's sexual identity.

Had Parr had any indication that there was an adult in the community who knew something about homosexuality and who would not immediately condemn his sister, perhaps he might have sought out that person. It would have been good if someone had had the knowledge to educate him about sexual orientation. For example, an informed guidance counselor or teacher might have been able to tell him that sexual orientation emerges for most people in early adolescence, without prior sexual experience, and is not a choice.

Evie and Patsy

Evie and Patsy will be discussed together as they are the only lesbian characters in the book and there are more similarities than differences in the interventions that might have benefited them.

Evie is presented as someone who accepts herself for who she is. She dresses and acts more like her father than her mother. Because the book is written from Parr's point of view, our sense of Evie is one step removed. Kerr allows us a closer look into Evie's world by having Evie share her poetry with Parr. Through her poetry we learn that Evie keeps a part of herself hidden from others, which she considers a "black-and-white life." After Evie begins to spend time with Patsy Duff, her poetry suggests that this encounter has awakened in her a desire to have more than a "black-and-white life." As Parr notes, "maybe there was something going on with her that was just bursting to come out" (25).

Evie begins to consider that she might be able to have a life that includes not only her family and farming, both of which she loves, but also a romantic relationship with someone who accepts her for who she is and with whom she shares a mutual attraction. But the reactions of others quickly let her see that she will not be able to stay in Duffton and have such a life. Patsy's father will not accept such a relationship between Patsy and Evie, and Evie does not wish to bring further embarrassment to her family. Even though her parents are more tolerant than Patsy's father is, they are far from accepting of her relationship with Patsy.

Returning to Erikson's theory, Evie does not have a social identity other than that afforded to her as a member of the farming community. Prior to her getting to know Patsy, who had been away at boarding school, Evie did not know other gay or lesbian adolescents or young adults. She lived with the constant nagging and matchmaking attempts of her mother. Most likely, Evie would have had difficulty even sooner had she not been comfortable with one major piece of her identity, that of being a farmer. She attempted (and until she met Patsy, successfully) to ignore other aspects of herself while she threw herself into her work. Although this compromise was satisfactory to others around Evie, eventually Evie's work was not enough for her.

Evie's choice is not an uncommon one for gay, lesbian, and bisexual young adults. Because of societal values against homosexuality, they must often make such difficult choices. Many move away from their hometowns to avoid embarrassing their families when they are seen publicly with same-gender girlfriends or boyfriends. Others, like Evie, leave rural areas where they feel that they cannot be understood and will always be outsiders. In addition, sexual minority youth frequently feel that they must choose between their sexual orientation and their religion. These are unfair and often unbearable choices. It is extremely painful to have to choose between aspects of oneself. For the most part, heterosexuals cannot even fathom such a choice—nor would they be asked to make such a choice.

What might have been helpful to Evie or Patsy, growing up in a small town and questioning their sexual identity? As with Parr, perhaps most helpful would have been firsthand knowledge of other gay, lesbian, or bisexual individuals. This opportunity probably existed for Patsy, who attended Appleman Academy, a boarding school outside of Duffton. Patsy may have met other nonheterosexual individuals, as well as having the benefit of a feminist perspective, as evidenced in the tale about her sweatshirt, which read "Appleperson Academy." Patsy's broader perspective may have been the result of encountering open-minded views, meeting others, or being exposed to books or videos with gay or lesbian characters. Thus, Kerr has appropriately drawn Patsy as the initiator in the relationship. Ironically, it is Evie who is blamed, especially by Mr. Duff, as the one who influenced or seduced Patsy. This form of denial is not an unusual response for parents who have learned that their child is nonheterosexual. In addition, as Parr's mother points out to him, because Evie "looks the part," she will be the one who is blamed. Patsy, who is described as looking very heterosexual, has been able to pass as a straight person, which Evie has not. This difference may have created variance in their levels of self-esteem, as Patsy was no doubt more popular and better able to fit in with her peers than was Evie.

Parr struggles to understand how stereotypes are relevant to his sister. His mother explains to him that Evie is a stereotype, that she is what everyone thinks a lesbian should be. What Parr's mother does not tell him is that if Evie were a gay male and fit that stereotype, her life could be much worse. Studies have repeatedly shown that people have more negative attitudes toward gay men than they do toward lesbians.

On the flip side, Patsy may have been subjected to a different type of pressure. Those individuals who are able to pass for heterosexual, along with those who are bisexual, are often pressured to choose heterosexuality. Parents such as Mr. Duff may understand that someone like Evie cannot change, but they are more confused by a daughter who looks heterosexual and who has dated males. Although bisexual individuals do have the capacity to be attracted to both the same and opposite gender, few people actually make a choice when it comes to falling in love.

What would be helpful to young people who are struggling to understand their sexual identity? First and foremost, what is needed from those who are significant to the individual is the assurance that they are still good people, that they will still be liked or loved, and that they will still be appreciated for themselves, regardless of their orientation. Unfortunately, such unconditional caring is not always available. Knowledge about sexuality and sexual identity development can also be very helpful.

Once Evie and Patsy move to a large urban area, such as New York City, their options for seeking assistance in dealing with their sexuality will increase dramatically. There will be a greater chance of finding a mental health professional who is gay-affirmative. Professional assistance may be necessary as they adjust to the multiple changes—and losses—they have experienced. At most colleges and universities, even in many rural areas, there are counseling centers that provide services to the students enrolled. Although the resources will vary from one school to another, college campuses often have support or therapy groups, offered through the counseling center, for sexual minority students. In addition, there are often student organizations, such as chapters of the Bisexual, Gay, and Lesbian Alliance (BiGALA), that provide opportunities for social, political, and/or educational activity.

Should Evie and Patsy have problems in their relationship, they are more likely, in a large city or on a college campus, to find a counselor or therapist who is familiar with some of the relationship difficulties that are particular to couples in stigmatized relationships. For example, many sexual minority couples are isolated from family and expect each other to be their sole source of love and companionship. Such expectations would place a heavy burden on any relationship. If one member of the couple is more comfortable with being "out" as a sexual minority than the other, this can cause conflict in the relationship.

Mr. and Mrs. Burrman

Like Parr, Evie's parents are impacted by Evie's choice to stop hiding her sexual identity. Although their gay and lesbian children embarrass many families, Evie's parents defend her to others. It is clear, however, that she has disappointed both of them. Patsy's decision to leave Duffton has major implications for the family's ability to pay off their loan and perhaps even remain farmers. Mrs. Burrman seems to long for a daughter who is more like her, with whom she can trade stories about clothing, sororities, and dating boys. Mr. Burrman is hurt and disappointed, as if he has lost his best friend.

Also like Parr, Mr. and Mrs. Burrman would have benefited from being able to talk with others who have family members who are gay and lesbian. Only one person in the novel, Sheriff Starr, made a clumsy attempt to offer support.

A Duffton chapter of the international organization Parents, Family, and Friends of Lesbians and Gays (PFLAG) might have proved most helpful to Evie's parents. PFLAG, as its name suggests, is made up of gay-affirmative individuals, most of whom are heterosexual family members of gays and lesbians. Most PFLAG chapters have monthly meetings, and members will often visit or speak on the telephone with parents who are struggling with the knowledge that their son or daughter is gay, lesbian, or bisexual.

PREVENTION

The Role of the School

What kinds of programs and resources could exist within the schools and surrounding community that might have contributed to an outcome different from the one portrayed in the novel? In some schools and communities across the country, creative yet realistic ideas are being tried.

Donovan Walling (1993) suggests that when examining a school's attitudes about gay teens, it is useful to think of a continuum from exclusive to inclusive. At the exclusive end, the school is clearly homophobic, and gay, lesbian, and bisexual students are verbally harassed or shunned. When such acts occur, teachers and administrators look the other way. At the more inclusive end of the continuum, there is an understanding that some students are questioning their sexual identity, and harassment is not tolerated. Prevention of hate crimes, as well as prevention of the acute isolation that both Parr and Evie experience, becomes increasingly possible in a more inclusive environment.

In schools, books such as *Deliver Us from Evie* and others (such as those listed in the recommended readings) can introduce young people to ideas and values that may be more gay-affirmative than those in their homes or their places of worship. Depending on the age of the students, such books may be better for independent reading than for assigned reading for a class. Including such books on suggested reading lists or in school libraries is another option.

Some high schools have groups for gay, lesbian, and bisexual students, and many such groups include allies, that is, supportive heterosexuals. No doubt Parr would have benefited from such a group. As one would expect, these groups are more common in large, urban areas. With the information explosion provided by the Internet and the World Wide Web, however, it is now possible for anyone with access to a computer to obtain information about sexual orientation or "chat" with others about issues of sexual orientation.

Walling (1993) lists five "attitude indicators" (20) that let gay and lesbian teens know that they can safely ask for help or talk about their feelings:

1. In their use of language, teachers and counselors do not assume that all teens are heterosexual.
2. Teachers speak out against harassment and humor at the expense of gays and lesbians.
3. Teachers openly discuss the contributions of gays and lesbians in a particular field.
4. Teachers and counselors have books or posters in their offices that show they are open to discussing gay and lesbian issues.
5. Counselors invite students whom they believe are struggling with issues of sexual orientation to come speak with them.

In addition to those students who are questioning their sexual identity, there is another group of students for whom this topic is relevant. These are the children who, like Parr, come from homes with gay, lesbian, or bisexual family members. Although the American family has been changing for some time, only within the last ten to fifteen years has homosexuality had a public family face. An estimated 14 million children have a lesbian or gay parent (Singer and Deschamps, 1994). It is crucial that teachers recognize the need for all children to have their families understood and respected.

The authors of this chapter are not naive about the pressures that can be brought to bear on teachers who try to raise controversial topics in their classrooms. Taking the lead with these topics can be especially difficult for those teachers who are gay, lesbian, bisexual, or transgender. Consequently, heterosexual professionals working in the schools play a vital role in making the schools a safer place for sexual minority youth. As members of the dominant culture, they are less likely to be accused of being "one of them." In the video documentary *It's Elementary*, one teacher pointed out that as a married woman with children, she felt much safer raising gay and lesbian issues in the classroom than did her gay colleagues. Even allies can be subject to harassment, and an assumption may be made that they must be gay as well or else would not take on such issues. For this reason, it is important that nondiscrimination policies be created. If students know that gay or lesbian teachers can be fired based on their orientation, it sends a clear message that the school is not safe for sexual minorities.

One of the biggest problems with addressing the topic of sexual orientation is that few professionals have received adequate training in this area. There are now many professionals who could be brought into schools for in-service instruction on this topic, and a wide array of written materials and videos are available for rental or purchase.

Why would schools be willing to take on such a controversial topic? Increasingly, educated people are aware of the burden that silence has placed on nonheterosexual individuals. As homosexuality comes out of its closet, more and more people realize that they know someone who is gay, lesbian, or bisexual. This increased visibility has put faces and names on what had been previously only a stereotype and an "illness." It is much easier for people to be against stereotypes and much harder for people to be against other human beings. Schools may also need to become more accepting for financial reasons. In 1996, Jeremy Nabozny won a lawsuit against his high school in Ashland, Wisconsin. He charged that the school district had not provided a safe environment for him to attend school. Despite the fact that he had reported numerous incidents of verbal and physical harassment from his peers, the school did nothing to protect him. Ashland officials were forced to pay Nabozny nearly $1 million in damages (*The Advocate*, January 21, 1997, 57–59). Sometimes, money talks.

The Role of the Community

In many communities, there is an organization or agency that functions as a hub, bringing together many gay-friendly individuals and organizations. Often this hub is a gay and lesbian community center, a building or some rented rooms that serve as a gathering place for gays, lesbians, bisexuals, and their allies. The center might serve any number of functions, including provision of a drop-in center for youth, a telephone hotline manned by volunteers, support groups, a lending library, rooms where various groups can hold organizational meetings, a referral list of gay-affirmative businesses and health care providers, or a local newsletter. Particularly for gay and lesbian teens, both a hotline and a drop-in center are very important for providing information and minimizing the isolation, which they often feel. Such public institutions carry a symbolic message as well: that being gay, lesbian, or bisexual is not something that must be hidden. Youth groups do not need to be housed in a gay and lesbian community center. Social service organizations, churches, health agencies, or other institutions may also sponsor such groups.

As mentioned previously, PFLAG is an important community resource. In addition to their primary function of providing support for family members, PFLAG chapters often participate in various advocacy and educational activities in the community. As parents, they have a powerful, impassioned voice that is often hard to ignore.

Religious organizations also have a powerful role to play. Within almost every organized religion there has been a move toward inclusion of sexual minorities. The Metropolitan Community Church, founded by the Reverend Troy Perry, was created specifically to respond to the varied religious and spiritual needs of gays, lesbians, and bisexuals. Other organizations have created offshoots, some officially recognized but most not, within specific denominations. These organizations include: Dignity (Catholic), Integrity (Episcopalian), Affirmation (Methodist), Friends for Gay and Lesbian Concerns (Quaker), and World Congress of Gay and Lesbian Jewish Organizations. Such religious organizations offer fellowship, solace, and spiritual support. Most important, they convey the message that one can be gay, lesbian, or bisexual and still be loved by, and maintain one's relationship with, God. Of course, a religious community does not have to be affiliated with one of these organizations to be gay-affirmative. Some sexual minority individuals have been lucky to find themselves accepted within their local church or synagogue.

The growing civil rights movement within the gay and lesbian community also serves a proactive function. Corporate policies and community ordinances that prohibit discrimination based on sexual orientation provide a legal framework in which to fight homophobia. Had such laws existed in Duffton, the sheriff would have had no business telling Evie to stay away from Patsy and, in fact, might have needed to warn Mr. Duffton that he could not harass Evie based on her orientation!

RECOMMENDED READINGS

Fiction

Bauer, Marion Dane. (Ed.). (1994). *Am I Blue?: Coming Out from the Silence*. New York: HarperCollins. 273 pp.(ISBN: 0–06–024253–1). MS.

The sixteen stories in this collection focus on the loneliness, confusion, pain, and joy that are part of growing up gay or lesbian. They also include characters who struggle to understand when they discover that friends are gay or lesbian.

Block, Francesca Lia. (1995). *Baby Be-Bop*. New York: HarperCollins. 106 pp. (ISBN: 0–06–024880–7). HS.

Dirk McDonald knows he does not fit the image Grandma Fifi has of him. He knows he doesn't like girls, and he waits for a way to change or a way to tell his grandma. In a night of magical fantasy, he learns that he and his way of loving are acceptable to himself and to Grandma Fifi.

Durant, Penny Raife. (1992). *When Heroes Die*. New York: Macmillan. 136 pp. (ISBN: 0–689–31764–6). MS.

To 12-year-old Gary, his uncle Rob is a hero, a surrogate father, and a best friend. When Uncle Rob gets very sick with AIDS, Gary worries that maybe he himself is gay, too, since he gets tongue-tied when he talks to girls. Gary suddenly has many questions and fears, but he finds answers and comfort in Uncle Rob.

Ecker, B. A. (1983). *Independence Day*. New York: Flare. 205 pp. (ISBN:0–380–82990–8). HS.

Although Mike has a girlfriend, plays soccer, and seems like many other 16-year-olds, he is filled with conflicting emotions. For some time he has known that he is "different," and he has come to realize that his feelings for his close friend Todd are more than just friendship. Now he wonders how his decision to announce those feelings to Todd on the Fourth of July will affect the rest of his life.

Futcher, Jane. (1981). *Crush*. Boston: Alyson. 248 pp. (ISBN: 1–55583–602–X). HS.

During her senior year at Huntington Hill, an exclusive girls' school, Jinx has a crush on the beautiful and popular Lexie. When the fascinating Lexie wants to be her friend, Jinx finally feels as if she belongs. Then, life becomes even more difficult for Jinx.

Hautzig, Deborah. (1989). *Hey, Dollface*. New York: Knopf. 151 pp. (ISBN: 0–394–82046–0). HS.

Fifteen-year-old Val Hoffman is a new student at Garfield School for Girls. She feels completely out of place until she meets Chloe Fox. The two girls become very close, sharing special secrets and much of their free time. Val eventually feels confused about the intensity of her feelings for Chloe. Could this be more than friendship?

Homes, A. M. (1989). *Jack*. New York: Macmillan. 220 pp. (ISBN: 0–02–744831–2). HS.

Jack is 14 when his father tells him that he is homosexual. Jack's mother and father are divorced, but Jack had been completely unaware that his father was gay. Jack thinks his best friend, Max, has a family that is just about perfect—until he discovers otherwise.

Kerr, M. E. (1997). *Hello, I Lied*. New York: HarperCollins. 171 pp. 171 pp. (ISBN: 0–06–027529–4). MS.

Seventeen-year-old Lang Penner spends the summer in the caretaker's cottage at Roundelay, the secluded, glitzy home of Ben Nevada, a famous but reclusive rock star. Lang meets Huguette, a teenager from France—and the mysterious Ben Nevada himself—before the summer is over.

Koertge, Ron. (1988). *The Arizona Kid*. Boston: Joy Street Books. 228 pp. (ISBN: 0–316–50101–8). MS.

Billy heads west to Arizona from Missouri to spend the summer with his uncle Wes, who is gay. In three months, Billy learns about himself and growing up. He experiences his first romance, finds his direction, and comes to understand his uncle. The frank language may offend some readers.

Scoppettone, Sandra. (1991). *Happy Endings Are All Alike*. Boston: Alyson. 202 pp. (ISBN: 1–55583–177–X). HS.

Jaret and Peggy are lovers. Jaret's mother knows of and accepts their lesbian relationship. Peggy's sister cannot accept it. After a brutal attack against Jaret, the girls, their families, and the town are all faced with handling Jaret and Peggy's relationship and different ideas on sexuality.

Nonfiction

Cohen, Susan, and Daniel Cohen. (1989). *When Someone You Know Is Gay*. New York: Evans. 162 pp. (ISBN: 0–87131–567–X). MS.

The authors discuss the topic of teenage homosexuality in a sensitive and straightforward way. Excerpts from interviews with gay teens illustrate the problems experienced by the teenage homosexual.

Evans, N. J., and V. A. Wall. (1991). *Beyond Tolerance: Gays, Lesbians and Bisexuals on Campus*. Alexandria, VA: American College Personnel Association. 232 pp. (ISBN: 1–555620–088–9). A.

This book, written for higher education officials, covers such issues as developmental models for sexual identity, becoming an ally, and addressing gay and lesbian issues in residence halls, fraternities, and sororities.

Fairchild, B., and N. Hayward. (1989). *Now That You Know*. San Diego: Harcourt Brace. 275 pp. (ISBN: 0–15–667601–X). HS.

This book is intended for gay, lesbian, and bisexual youth to give to their parents or other family members after disclosing their sexual orientation. This is an important resource for young people who are not yet able to answer many of their family's questions related to sexual identity.

Fricke, Aaron. (1981). *Reflections of a Rock Lobster: A Story about Growing Up Gay*. Boston: Alyson. 116 pp. (ISBN: 0–932870–09–0). HS.

In this autobiographical novel, a young man tells of coming to terms with his gay feelings and how he developed the strength of spirit to challenge school authorities.

Harbeck, K. M. (1992). *Coming Out of the Classroom Closet: Gay and Lesbian Students, Teachers and Curricula*. New York: Harrington Park. 271 pp. (ISBN: 1–56023–013–4). HS.

This is a collection of essays geared toward individuals interested in improving the climate for lesbian and gay persons in our schools, colleges, and universities.

Kranz, Rachel. (1992). *Straight Talk about Prejudice*. New York: Facts On File. 124 pp. (ISBN): 0–8160–2488–X). HS.

Although this book deals with many forms of prejudice, the chapter on prejudice against homosexuals is exceptional. Chapter 4 is structured around a stereotype- and myth-awareness test about homosexuality.

Kuklin, Susan. (1993). *Speaking Out: Teenagers Take on Race, Sex, and Identity*. New York: Putnam. 165 pp. (ISBN: 0–399–22532–3). HS.

Susan Kuklin asked a group of people to discuss prejudice, race, sexuality, and being different. When the students were given the chance to talk for themselves, they clearly showed that their feelings were the same—it hurts to be labeled.

Langone, John. (1993). *Spreading Poison: A Book about Racism and Prejudice*. Boston: Little, Brown. 178 pp. (ISBN: 0–316–51410–1). HS.

John Langone examines various myths and stereotypes surrounding racial bigotry, religious persecution, and homosexuality, along with historical and social events that fostered them.

Monette, Paul. (1988). *Borrowed Time: An AIDS Memoir*. San Diego: Harcourt Brace. 342 pp. (ISBN: 0–15–113598–3). HS.

Author, poet, and playwright Paul Monette's memoir of the death of his male companion from AIDS. This is a story of devotion, sacrifice, and love, and anger at modern medicine's lack of effective weapons for fighting the ailment.

Rench, Janice E. (1990). *Understanding Sexual Identity: A Book for Gay Teens and Their Friends*. Minneapolis: Lerner. 56 pp. (ISBN: 0–8225–0044–2). MS.

The author's goal is to dispel some of the myths about gay and lesbian people and to help all readers, regardless of their sexual orientation, become more comfortable with differences.

REFERENCES

Anderson, J. D. (1997). "Supporting the Invisible Minority." *Educational Leadership* 54 (7): 65–68.

Cass, V. C. (1979). "Homosexuality Identity Formation: A Theoretical Model." *Journal of Homosexuality* 4: 219–235.

Coleman, E. (1982). "Developmental Stages of the Coming-out Process." In W. Paul, J. D. Weinrick, J. Gonsiorek, and M. E. Hotvedt (Eds.), *Homosexuality: Social, Psychological and Biological Issues*, Beverly Hills, CA: Sage, 31–43.

Erikson, E. (1963). *Childhood and Society*. New York: Norton.

Harbeck, K. M. (1992). *Coming Out of the Classroom Closet: Gay and Lesbian Students, Teachers and Curricula*. New York: Harrington Park.

It's Elementary: Talking about Gay Issues in School. (1996). Directed by Debra Chasnoff. Produced by Helen S. Cohen and Debra Chasnoff. San Francisco, CA: Women's Educational Media.

Kerr, M. E. (1994). *Deliver Us from Evie*. New York: HarperCollins.

Remafedi, G. (1994). *Death by Denial*. Boston: Alyson.

Singer, B. L., and D. Deschamps. (1994). *Gay and Lesbian Stats*. New York: New Press.

Troiden, R. R. (1979). "Becoming Homosexual; A Model of Gay Identity Acquisition." *Psychiatry* 42: 362–373.

Walling, D. R. (1993). *Gay Teens at Risk*. Bloomington, IN: Phi Delta Kappa Educational Foundation.

CHAPTER 4

Identity through Intimacy: Jenny Davis's *Sex Education*

Marie Hardenbrook, Patti Mahoney, Jennifer Khera, and Margaret Goldman

INTRODUCTION

> I helped her out of the nightgown very slowly, first pulling her arms out and then drawing the nightgown carefully over her head. What I saw stunned me. She was covered with bruises. Everywhere. Some were old and greenish yellow. Some, most, were fairly fresh, black and ugly blue. Two places on her arms were raw red and still swelling. "He's beating you," I gasped. "Maggie he's beating you." (Davis, 1995, 135)

At least 2 to 4 million women each year are physically abused, and as many as 60% of married couples have experienced violence sometime during their marriage, according to the surgeon general's report, *A Medical Response to Domestic Violence* (Novello, 1992). Karen Hanson, in "Gendered Violence: Examining Education's Role" (1995), cites the work of Nancy Worcester on adolescent battering as well as Barrie Levy's research on dating violence to support her conclusion that there are "significant similarities between adult battering relationships and those of adolescents" (5). More than one in ten adolescents reported violence in their dating relationships (Levy, 1998). Four out of five students in an American Association of University Women Educational Foundation study, *Hostile Hallways* (1993), stated they had been harassed.

Teenagers today need positive models for healthy intimate relationships; they also need the support of caring adults as they search for the answers to their questions:

Who am I as a girl or boy?

When am I ready to have sex?

Am I sexually desirable if I do not have a perfect body?

What does having sex really mean?

What does sex have to do with intimacy?

Who am I in the relationship?

The National Longitudinal Study on Adolescent Health, a study of more than ninety thousand adolescents in the United States, confirmed that emotional connectedness to home and school were the most critical protective factors of adolescents against emotional distress, suicide, violence, substance abuse, and sexual behaviors (Resnick, 1997). According to young adult writer Shelly Stoehr (1997), teens resist discussion with adults of topics concerning sex and drugs; books allow for discussion of those same issues in a "non-threatening manner" (5). Jenny Davis's book *Sex Education* (1995) is a gutsy coming-of-age novel that deals frankly with adolescent curiosity about and involvement with sex as well as dealing with the issues of teenage pregnancy, body image, domestic violence, and death. *Sex Education* could be the story of any teenager.

SYNOPSIS

Livvie is 14 years old and is once again a new kid in school. Her father's job with IBM has made it necessary for the family to move six different times. Knowing she will not stay in the same school very long, Livvie chooses not to participate in group activities such as clubs or sports; all of her activities are solitary ones such as walking and reading. In Mrs. Fulton's Biology 200 class she meets David, a 15-year-old boy born and raised in High Ridge. They share a love for walking and become partners in Mrs. Fulton's sex education project. Mrs. Fulton has a mission and, as Livvie senses, "she was like a scientist trying out a new hypothesis" (22). Through her summer job analyzing blood and urine specimens, Mrs. Fulton observes firsthand the emotional trauma facing pregnant teenagers. She believes it is her moral obligation to teach sex education.

Mrs. Fulton gives her students several projects. One, the mirror project, asks students to look at themselves naked in the mirror and to accept themselves completely. Another project involves caring about someone else, someone they do not know. David and Livvie become partners in the caring project by adopting a pregnant neighbor, Maggie Parker. When Maggie and her husband, Dean, move in, Maggie faints in front of her new house. The whole neighborhood, including David and Livvie, come to her rescue and help the new neighbors move into their house. Dean seems remote and unfriendly. He posts "Do Not Disturb" and "No Trespassing" signs on their front lawn. Unaware of their true meaning, Livvie and David attribute the signs to Mr. Parker's desire to protect his wife's health, and they continue to visit Maggie while Dean Parker is at work. Besides her inability to keep food down, Maggie is also dealing with a problem created by the highway department's blasting for a new roadway. When an insurance investigator visits and inspects a crack in the house's foundation, Maggie is buoyed by the promise of insurance compensation that will allow her to fix up her house. Livvie and David's visits with Maggie often involve discussing plans for the house. Maggie invites David and Livvie to her husband's Christmas office party, which the Parkers are hosting. When Livvie and David witness Dean Parker being inappropriately friendly with another woman, Dean becomes hostile, and Maggie becomes withdrawn and noncommunicative.

"There were times," Livvie says of her relationship with David, that "we thought only of ourselves and each other, of the we that we were forming, becoming" (95). Although they were from very different circumstances, Livvie muses, "we were the same inside" (27). Unlike Livvie's family, David had lived in High Ridge his entire life. Marie, his adoptive mother, is a midwife who helped David's teenage mother, Rachel, give birth. Rachel left David for Marie to raise. Livvie contrasts David's relationship with Marie, which is one of friendship, with her distant relationship with her parents, whom Livvie sees as adult figures more concerned with the superficialities of life.

As Maggie becomes more withdrawn and indicates that she is doing too poorly to have visitors, Livvie and David's relationship grows more sexual. Livvie reflects that it is perhaps because they no longer have anywhere to direct their excess energy and caring. Livvie and David never actually have sex, and they never have the chance to live out their relationship. After hearing that Maggie has given birth to a boy, David and Livvie visit her. Getting no response at the door, they hear Maggie calling them. After entering the house, they find Maggie in bed, lying in her own feces, with the baby by her side. Confronting the horrible truth that Maggie is abused, Livvie helps her get ready to leave while David attempts to divert Dean Parker, who has come home unexpectedly.

In an angry confrontation on the front porch, Dean pushes David down the icy stairs. David's neck snaps, and he falls dead at Livvie's feet. Unable to deal with the loss of David, Livvie becomes catatonic and is subsequently hospitalized in a psychiatric facility. Readers first meet Livvie as she recalls her journey of love and loss.

ANALYSIS

Donelson and Nilsen point out in *Literature for Today's Young Adults* (1997): "Often the difference in the life span between two books that are equally well written from a literary standpoint is that the ephemeral book fails to touch kids where they live, whereas the long-lasting book treats experiences that are psychologically important to young people" (34).

Girls today will identify with Livvie's description of the thrill of her first kiss, David's arousal of her sexual feelings, and her pride at being known as David's girl. "When it happened," she says, "I knew I had been waiting for it all my life" (37). They will identify, too, with Livvie's admission that the gap between her feelings for David and her feelings for the Parkers "was so big as to be an embarrassment" (60). Livvie's real interest was not in the project as much as it was in being with David.

Livvie and David's relationship is what most girls want for themselves: a relationship based on equality and mutual caring. The adult relationship of Maggie with Dean is destructive and denigrating and provides a striking contrast. The crack in the foundation of Maggie's house symbolizes a fault in the foundation of her marriage. Livvie observes David's thoughtfulness in caring for Maggie and concern while Dean's efforts are noticeably absent. David comments that he finds it difficult to understand a husband who does not care for his wife, and Livvie's thoughts dwell on what it would be like to be married to a man as caring and sensitive as David.

The messages of the book are critical ones for teens: develop your own self-identity; sexual maturity will take time; sex is part of a loving, caring relationship; your choices regarding when to have sex and with whom can have significant consequences. Unfortunately, consequences of having loving or sexual relationships are negative for the main characters. Maggie is abused, Livvie is catatonic, David is dead, and Mrs. Fulton is guilt ridden. This is a much different message from the message of popular culture, which glamorizes sexual exploitation and conquest.

THERAPY AND COUNSELING FOR LIVVIE AND DAVID: A ROUNDTABLE DISCUSSION BETWEEN THE AUTHORS

Hardenbrook: Parental and school connectedness is an important factor in deterring young adults from engaging in unhealthy risk taking. In Davis's novel we know that David is close to his adoptive mother, Marie, but what about Livvie's relationship with her parents?

Mahoney: I would call her relationship with her parents far more normal than David and Marie's relationship. Her parents are watching her, and she wants to be left alone.

Hardenbrook: And, of course, all her energies are tied up with David. Do you see similar relationships with the students you counsel? Is this kind of relationship realistic?

Mahoney: I saw this part of the book as very unrealistic. I do not see adolescents as capable of that kind of relationship. I see David and Livvie's relationship as a rather mature relationship, a relationship more characteristic of perhaps 24-year-olds, but not 14-year-olds.

Khera: Yes, I see a lot of girls at 15 with the marriage dream.

Hardenbrook: Livvie has some of that marriage dream. Several times in the book she wonders what it would be like to be David's wife, and she contrasts her ideal life with David against the dread that Maggie is experiencing in her marriage.

Goldman: Jennifer and I teach abuse prevention through respect education. We absolutely agree that books allow for discussion of topics relevant to youth in a nonthreatening manner and absolutely advocate using books to educate about social issues. In fact, this is one of the ways in which we implement our programs. In reviewing the book *Sex Education*, we would approach it as if we were thinking about it as one of our recommended books. For example, I believe that a positive relationship between parents and teens is essential, so I would have the students examine the characteristics of Livvie and David's relationship with their parents. I would ask the students characteristics of a good friendship and how they differ, if they do, from the characteristics of a loving couple's relationship. From this I would focus on what characteristics best describe respect, and I would ask the students to write or discuss what respect for oneself means. Ultimately, I would hope to discuss that aspect of respect for self which translates into planning for good things to happen in one's life, such as goals and plans for achieving those goals. At some point I would question, given the risks, how wise it is to have sex at 14.

Khera: Right. I would phrase questions for discussion that would focus on the development of a sense of self. *Sex Education* is understandably a popular book among teens. It depicts a young woman's romanticized and idealized view of love, which, I believe, is rare if not impossible to experience in that age group. It is what women long for at any age, but I think it is unrealistic. According to a recent study, seventy percent of females are sexually active by age 18. I wonder how many of those young women had sex because they were in love like Livvie and how many were coerced or got drunk and had sex, and then just thought, "Oh well, I've already done it once. It doesn't matter." I think I would focus on what consent looks like and what young women want for themselves.

Goldman: With regard to respect for self, I would say that I did like the exercise in the book in which the teacher had the students look at themselves naked in the mirror and accept themselves completely. Our society demands so much of us physically. Women can't be thin enough, and men should be strong and athletic. I would use this chance to focus on stereotypes and how harmful they can be to all of us. One exercise that I might suggest is to have the students bring in pictures from popular magazines or have them monitor their favorite TV shows and identify how the media, our culture, depicts the ideal male or female.

Khera: Let's talk about the teacher. Teachers have such an opportunity to play a significant role in young people's lives. I would ask the students what Mrs. Fulton does well and where she fails. I think this teacher is irresponsible. She urges her students to care for someone else as a means of learning how to care for oneself, without talking about what caring means. And she should have intervened when Livvie and David told her about the Parkers. Marie should have done something as well. That Livvie and David are not at all suspicious that abuse exists with the Parkers indicates how young they are. I would use this opportunity to discuss dating violence and domestic abuse.

Hardenbrook: I agree! Moreover, I believe as parents and educators, we need to reexamine our role in perpetuating societal stereotypes and the power dynamics associated with gendered roles. Patti, if Livvie came to see you and told you that she and David had a mature relationship and she was trying to decide whether or not to have sex with him, what would you have said?

Mahoney: I would have said, "I can't give you an answer; only you know that answer." But what I would be thinking is, "Developmentally, I know you are not capable of thinking in those terms."

Hardenbrook: Shaughnessy and Shakeby state in their article on adolescent emotional intimacy that adolescents do not have the required skills to be emotionally intimate and therefore rely on physical intimacy. So you think Livvie was not ready?

Mahoney: Absolutely not. You have to have two wholes to mutually give yourself to each other. The primary developmental task of adolescence is identity. Adolescents do not know who they are. You cannot be intimate with another person until you know what you are sharing. You have to have this level of self-knowledge. I honestly do not believe most adolescents are ready, particularly now, with our attitudes about education and dependency on parents. I have had teenage boys come into my office and say with great sincerity that they could not have sex with certain girls because they are friends! And I say, "Okay, help me on this."

Hardenbrook: So adolescent boys separate sex from friendship?

Mahoney: Yes! With girls, the feelings are there, but it's almost pure fantasy the way they view marriage and romance at this point in their lives. Their emotions are not reality based at all. And unless they have relationships modeled by their parents, their notion of romance is based on their emotional response to, let's say, a movie like *Titanic*, where the girls go and cry their eyes out.

Hardenbrook: Erikson's definition of the adolescent period as a time of identity development—is this the psychological basis for Livvie and David not being ready for this mature relationship?

Mahoney: Yes, Erikson outlined eight developmental stages. The fifth stage, the adolescent period, is not how we define it today. I would say adolescence could even be extended, in some cases, to as late as 25. Economically, we have supported our children in trying this or that, but not in fully developing their own identity separate from their parents. So their ability to be truly intimate with another is delayed. After developing a sense of self that is stable and consistent, then an individual is ready for the sixth stage, which involves the acquired skill of intimacy.

Goldman: Part of the extension of adolescence is because we as parents are more allowing of our children's wishes to do the off-the-wall kinds of things they might want to do. When my generation was growing up, you went to college and you were going to be a teacher or a nurse or whatever; and you knew once you got out of college, you had to do something that made money. We made a living. And now kids talk about finding their passion. They are given more license to find themselves. When I was a young adult, society really did not condone exploring. We didn't talk about finding our passion.

Hardenbrook: I agree we have extended the adolescent period. One thought I had about Livvie's focus on her relationship with David rather than setting personal goals toward developing other parts of her life is based on a discussion I had with the director of our teenage parenting program. This woman had directed the program for over twenty years and was the mother of two grown daughters. I asked her, "If you could identify one characteristic of a girl who enters the teen pregnancy program, what would it be?" I will never forget her answer. She said, "A girl without a plan." Given this, if Livvie, being all of 14, came to me and said she had a mature relationship with David and wanted to have sex with him and marry him, I would be inclined to suggest that she needed to be thinking about what she was going to be doing with the rest of her life. Is this how you would handle it?

Mahoney: Not really, because that would be giving advice. A functional analysis approach would be more psychologically appropriate. What I would ask Livvie to think about is what she is going to get out of the relationship. In developing this connection, is she recreating the emotional connection that she gave up with her family? And if this is what she is doing, is there a better way to do it? I would ask her to weigh the pros and cons of what she is proposing to do. What are the risks? Pregnancy, heartbreak, a sexually transmitted disease . . . I would ask, "What are you looking for?"

Hardenbrook: If I could be 14 again, in answer to your question "What are you looking for?" I would say, "I want someone to just love me." Then what would you say?

Mahoney: Well, I would go right back to risk again. What risks are you taking, and can you get the same thing without risks?

Hardenbrook: Mrs. Fulton did her job well. Livvie rattles off all the sexual parts of the body as well as the sexually related diseases. Yet, she still wants to have sex with David. What about David? Do boys come and talk to you about having sex?

Mahoney: Yes, they do, but it is usually after the fact. Boys often go through terrible guilt and fear about the consequences. Boys who are sexually active, at times, are dealing with a lack of impulse control, rather than the desire to be connected to another person, and the next thing they know, the girl is pregnant.

Hardenbrook: Another issue in the book that perplexes me is that David and Livvie do not pick up the warnings that perhaps the situation at the Parker home is dangerous. When they talk with their teacher and with Marie, both adults seem to indicate that there is trouble, but neither one goes so far as to say "Pay attention" or "Stay away."

Mahoney: The teacher was at fault because she should have known that there was something there that was of concern.

Khera: I think it is a good book for parents to read because it can show parents, if they are the type of family that doesn't talk about these things, what teens are thinking about, and it can be a red flag to parents to find out what their teens are doing. Where are they going? How much time are they spending alone?

Hardenbrook: Davis's portrayal of Maggie was quite accurate from what I know of abuse. She was trapped in the cycle of abuse.

Mahoney: She was right there.

Hardenbrook: The abuse situation brings up the esteem issue, the importance of a healthy self-esteem. Mindy Bingham's book *Things Will Be Different for My Daughter* cites feminist theorists who maintain that Erikson's work was primarily with males. They believe that females vacillate between intimacy and identity. As a result, if self-identity is fragile when they form an intimate relationship, they tend to define themselves by the relationship. This is what I saw happening to both Livvie and Maggie.

Mahoney: Yes, and it doesn't just happen to adolescent females!

Hardenbrook: My concern is that boys will not read *Sex Education*. As a high school librarian, I do not see boys reading about romance. Robert Lipsyte, an author of young adult literature, says boys are afraid to read certain books because the culture, mostly through peer pressure, doesn't allow it. He believes boys need to learn what girls already know: that a book allows you to explore and find out what life's all about. He contends boys need to know about relationships and being friends, not just with other boys, but with girls, too. This point brings us back to the negative influence of gender stereotypes. Boys feel pressure to be strong and tough, and reading about relationships is not a masculine activity.

CONCLUSION

Literacy autobiographies (autobiographies that discuss the importance of books in personal development and growth) suggest that books form almost a support system during life events (Bean and Readance, 1995). Studies suggest that adults who recall the importance of reading in their lives usually associate books with an emotional connection to caring, loving adults. Davis's book *Sex Education* and others like it can provide the emotional connection necessary for adolescents to receive adult support during their search for sexual identity.

RECOMMENDED READINGS

Fiction

Abraham, Pearl. (1995). *The Romance Reader*. Berkeley, CA: Riverhead. 296 pp. (ISBN: 1–573–22–548–7). MS, HS.

The oldest of seven children in an Orthodox Jewish family, Rachel is the "romance reader" of the title. She is addicted to the romance fiction of the drugstore, and she fantasizes about her romantic adventures. Her biggest challenge is to deal with her parents' plan for her arranged marriage.

Barrett, Elizabeth. (1994). *Free Fall*. New York: HarperCollins. 249 pp. (ISBN: 0–06–024465–8). HS.

Sent to her grandmother for the summer because of her parents' failing marriage, 17-year-old Ginnie struggles with the ups and downs of her own romantic relationship.

Bertrand, Diane Gonzales. (1995). *Sweet Fifteen*. Houston: Arte. 224 pp. (ISBN: 1–558–85184–4). MS, HS.

As Stephanie's fifteenth birthday approaches, her celebration is shadowed by the recent death of her domineering father. Stephanie comes to terms with her own identity as a female in a traditional Hispanic home as she seeks answers about her future in relationships.

Blume, Judy. (1975). *Forever*. New York: Bradbury. 199 pp. (ISBN: 0–027–11030–3). HS.

When Katherine meets and falls in love with Michael, she feels it will be forever. This novel focuses on first love, losing one's virginity, and family relationships.

Bridgers, Sue Ellen. (1998). *Permanent Connections*. New York: Replica. 272 pp. (ISBN: 0–735–10043–8). HS.

Seventeen-year-old Rob finds himself in new relationships with friends and family when he is forced to spend time in his father's small hometown in the mountains.

Christiansen, C. B. (1995). *I See the Moon*. New York: Atheneum. 115 pp. (ISBN: 0–689–31928–2). HS.

Looking forward to being an aunt, 12-year-old Bitte is thrilled that her 15-year-old sister Kari is having a baby. Bitte learns more about the complexity of love as she watches her sister struggle with the decision about her baby's future.

Cole, Shelia. (1995). *What Kind of Love?: The Diary of a Pregnant Teenager*. New York: Lothrop, Lee & Shepard. 192 pp. (ISBN: 0–688–12848–3). HS.

Valerie finds herself pregnant and must decide whether to give up her desire to be a classical musician or to give up the baby.

Cormier, Robert. (1997). *Tenderness*. New York: Delacorte. 249 pp. (ISBN: 0–385–32286–0). HS.

Eighteen-year-old Eric Poole, recently released from prison for the murder of his parents, and Lori, a 15-year-old runaway, both seek "tenderness."

Creech, Sharon. (1995). *Absolutely Normal Chaos*. New York: HarperCrest. 230 pp. (ISBN: 0–060–26992–8). HS.

Mary Lou Finney reluctantly begins writing a journal as a summer project for school. She chronicles her experiences with first love, death, friendship, and family.

Kaye, Geraldine. (1992). *Someone Else's Baby*. New York: Hyperion. 138 pp. (ISBN: 1–56292–149–0). HS.

As a result of a sexual encounter after having too much to drink at a party, 17-year-old Terry is pregnant and single. Told through her journal, the story reveals Terry's confusion and loneliness.

Nonfiction

Bell, Ruth. (1998). *Changing Bodies, Changing Lives: A Book for Teens on Sex and Relationships*. New York: New York Times. 320 pp. (ISBN: 0–8129–2990–X). MS. HS.

A new and updated version of a title popular with teens that discusses a wide variety of topics of interest to teens, including birth control, AIDS, teen pregnancy, relationships, and substance abuse.

Bode, Janet. (1997). *Trust and Betrayal: Real-life Stories of Friends and Enemies*. New York: Delacorte. 176 pp. (ISBN: 0–440–22035–1). HS.

Discusses peer relationships in the context of pregnancy, sexual harassment, disability, and a wide range of other issues.

Brumberg, Joan Jacobs. (1997). *The Body Project: An Intimate History of American Girls*. New York: Random House. 304 pp. (ISBN: 0–679–40297–7). HS

This book discusses in a historical context the evolution of the body image as self-identity for girls.

Caron, Ann F. (1995). *Strong Mothers, Strong Sons: Raising the Next Generation of Men*. New York: Harper Perennial. 336 pp. (ISBN: 0–060–97648–9). HS, A.

Focusing on the challenge of raising sons, this book highlights the issues of violence, sexuality, and attitudes toward women.

Carroll, Rebecca, and Ntozake Shange. (1997). *Sugar in the Raw: Voices of Young Black Girls in America*. New York: Crown. 144 pp. (ISBN: 0–517–88497–6). HS.

Carroll interviewed fifty young black women and chose fifteen stories to present in this volume of profiles of young black women between the ages of 11 and 20. They reflect on their future as black women and share their thoughts on topics such as race, sex, and gender.

Chailet, Donna. (1998). *Staying Safe at Home*. Get Prepared Library of Violence Prevention for Young Women. New York: Rosen. 64 pp. (ISBN: 0–8239–2740–7). MS, HS.

Information for young women on self-defense and protection from threats such as stalkers and domestic violence.

Dee, Catherine. (1997). *The Girls' Guide to Life: How to Take Charge of the Issues That Affect You*. New York: Little, Brown. 247 pp. (ISBN: 0–316–17952–3). MS.

Using a teen-magazine style, this handbook addresses gender stereotypes and advises girls on how to recognize and handle bias. The "Things to Do" chapter as well as first-person narratives from women such as Gloria Steinem and Maya Angelou make this a guide for the contemporary young woman.

Gay, Kathlyn. (1995). *Rights and Respect: What You Need to Know about Gender Bias and Sexual Harassment*. Brookfield, CT: Millbrook. 128 pp. (ISBN: 1–56294–493–2). HS.

Excellent discussion of the issues related to gender bias and harassment in the workplace and at school.

Hicks, John. (1996). *Dating Violence: True Stories of Hurt and Hope*. Brookfield, CT: Millbrook. 112 pp. (ISBN: 1–562–94654–4). HS.

Interviews with abusers and victims provide the basis for discussion of the characteristics of abusive relationships and the importance of resolving conflicts.

McCoy, K., and C. Wibbelsman. (1996). *Life Happens: A Teenager's Guide to Friends, Failure, Sexuality, Love, Rejection, Addiction, Peer Pressure, Families, Loss, Depression, Change, and Other Challenges*. New York: Perigee. 224 pp. (ISBN: 0–339–51987–4). HS.

The authors of *The New Teenage Body Book* (1992) provide a comprehensive support manual to help teens deal with the problems of living in a complex society.

REFERENCES

Bean, T. W., and J. Readance. (1995). "A Comparative Study of Content Area Literacy Students' Attitudes toward Reading through Autobiography Analysis." *Yearbook of the National Reading Conference* 44: 325–333.

Bingham, Mindy, and S. Stryker. (1995). *Things Will Be Different for My Daughter.* New York: Penguin.

Davis, Jenny. (1995). *Sex Education.* New York: Dell.

Donelson, K., and A. P. Nilsen. (1997) *Literature for Today's Young Adults.* New York: Addison-Wesley.

Hanson, K. (1995). "Gendered Violence: Examining Education's Role." *Center for Equity and Diversity Working Paper 4.* Newton, MA: Educational Development Center.

Hostile Hallways: The AAUW Survey on Sexual Harassment in America's Schools. (1993). Commissioned by the American Association of University Women Educational Foundation. Researched by Harris/Scholastic Research. Washington, DC: The Foundation.

Kaywell, Joan F. (1993). *Adolescents at Risk: A Guide to Fiction and Nonfiction for Young Adults, Parents, and Professionals.* Westport, CT: Greenwood.

Levy, Barrie. (1998). *Dating Violence: Young Women in Danger,* 2nd ed. Seattle: Seal.

Novello, Antonio, M. D. (1992). "From the Surgeon General, U.S. Public Health Service, a Medical Response to Domestic Violence." *Journal of the American Medical Association* 267 (23): 3132.

Resnick, M., P. S. Bearman, R. W. Blum, and K. E. Bauman. (1997). "Protecting Adolescents from Harm: Findings from the National Longitudinal Study on Adolescent Health." *Journal of the American Medical Association* 278 (10): 823–832.

Stoehr, Shelly. (1997). "Controversial Issues in the Lives of Contemporary Young Adults." *The ALAN Review* 24 (2): 3–5.

CHAPTER 5

Identity through Self-Awareness: Kathryn Lasky's *Memoirs of a Bookbat*

Patricia A. Crawford and Rosaria C. Upchurch

> A pebble on a sandy beach can change the course of a river, a tiny dewdrop can warp a giant oak forever.
>
> —Author unknown

We expect that our lives will be impacted by our circumstances. Be they positive or negative, joyful or tragic, we know that looming rites of passage and other key events will not only leave their marks, but will also have the potential to transform our worlds in significant ways. However, the driving forces that ultimately change our life course and perspective often lie not so much in the big events, but rather in the small, seemingly insignificant happenings of our daily experiences. Often, we operate in a type of survival mode, navigating each hurdle that comes our way and developing strategies to cope with all that life has to offer. Only with time, perspective, and a growing sense of self can we come to better understand the cumulative impact that these passing events have had on our lives and personal development. Only then can we come to a point of decision, a turning point where we suddenly realize that we must take control of our life circumstances, lest they take control of our very sense of being.

SYNOPSIS

Such is the case for Harper Jessup, Kathryn Lasky's delightful, resilient, and complex protagonist in *Memoirs of a Bookbat* (1994). As the story opens, Harper is a young girl who has already lived a life full of ups and downs and who is learning to cope with the roars of her life circumstances, as well as with the whispers of her relationships. By the age of 8, she already sees herself as a caregiver. When her family experiences financial duress, she desperately longs to make things better for them. When her parents fight, she strives to protect her younger sister from the conflict. And when her mother is bleeding and hurt, victimized by her father's abuse, Harper tries desperately to pick up the pieces of life in both a literal and figurative way. *Memoirs of a Bookbat* is the story of Harper's growing awareness of the many fragments in her life and her longing for a sense of wholeness, both as a member of her family and as an individual.

As *Memoirs of a Bookbat* begins, 14-year-old Harper finds herself staring out of the window of a cross-country bus, heading for a place of hoped-for sanity. As she speeds away from her parents' life and control, she reflects back on the many twists and turns that have brought her to this point.

Younger Days, Younger Ways

From all appearances, Harper's early childhood was rather unremarkable. Surrounded by her parents, Hank and Beth, and her younger sister, Weesie, Harper began her life in a neat and tidy home surrounded by "a little patch of yard" (7). However, everything seems to change when her family experiences financial problems. Trouble abounds, and the family is forced to leave their modest home and move into a tiny trailer. At first, Harper is enchanted with the idea of living in a house on wheels, envisioning a home that rolls from one wonderful, exciting experience to another. However, her hopes are quickly dashed as trailer life turns out to be less of a rolling adventure and more of a dank, shoebox-like existence that puts them on the outskirts of town, as well as on the margins of mainstream life. It soon appears that the Jessups' home, and their dreams, will remain firmly planted in a trailer park existence that is punctuated only by her father's occasional eruptions of anger.

As she navigates a sea of turbulent circumstances, Harper learns to pay careful attention to her parents' relationship and their personal interactions. She knows her parents and their routines so well that she is able to anticipate the roles that they will each play, as well as the nuances that characterize their interactions. For example, she knows that when her father lashes out in anger, her mother will quietly and gently try to soothe him. This will only anger her father further, until he feels compelled to storm out of their tiny, cramped home, leaving her mother in tears and Harper groping for an appropriate response. With this pattern so well established, Harper is caught off guard one day when her mother expresses a new sense of resolve and takes a more assertive stand. Confronted with the news that her husband has just lost his job once and for all, her mother does not try to coddle or cajole, nor does she smooth or smother. Instead, she simply announces that she and her husband will be going out for the evening; they will be going to church.

Finding Religion

Religion had never played a big role in the life of the Jessup family. At least it hadn't until that night when her parents went to church, where they lay hold of some hope for the first time in a very long while.

Harper noticed the change from the minute her parents walked in the door from church. Something had happened in the last few hours. When her parents returned from the service, they looked happier and healthier than they had before. Her mother appeared to be refreshed, and her father no longer seemed to be angry about losing his job. The change not only affected her parents as individuals but also as a couple. They returned from the service with a new sense of one another. And although Harper didn't quite know what had happened at that church meeting, she knew that she liked it because it had somehow bound them as a family.

The changes that Harper sensed that first night were only the beginning. In the days ahead, her parents began to go to church more and more. They joined Bible studies and went to nightly prayer meetings. Her mother baked for special events, and her father began to do repair work around the church building. Eventually, they came to do much more than attend events; they came to belong. As Harper tries to make sense of all the changes in her parents' world, she glimpses the power and impact of social group membership, noting:

> I guess the easy answer to their happiness is that they had found God. But it was different than that, really. I'm not sure whether they'd actually lost God before, anyway. I think it was like they found a group of people to be with and talk to. It might have been the first time they had friends, for all I know. (20)

In spite of her youth, Harper realizes that experiencing a sense of belonging and being part of a group bigger than oneself can make all the difference. And, at least in the beginning, these differences were good ones.

Into the Fold

Church brought a whole array of changes to the Jessups' world. The first change occurred when church came into their home in the form of regular and lengthy visits from well-meaning members. These new friends continuously and enthusiastically share their views on everything from the spirituality of family life to the necessity of strict parenting, firm discipline, and sheltering one's children from governmental intervention, inappropriate schooling, and other forms of spiritual attack. For her part, Harper continues to be a "very obedient child" (38) who loves to learn and read, and who finds tremendous solace in the world of books. Although Beth views Harper as being "rather bookish" (22), she is very proud of her daughter's behavior and boasts to her new church friends, "I declare, I don't think I've ever heard Harper talk back in her life" (38).

Eventually, Harper comes to experience a nagging sense of ambivalence about the new church friends and the resulting changes in their home life. On one hand, she is relieved to see her parents happily engaged with new acquaintances. And, as her parents' viewpoint on moral and spiritual issues becomes more narrow, she finds a growing sense of confidence in their protective care. When Beth passionately declares, "We know what is best for our children. . . . No government is going to love my daughters the way that I love them" (38), Harper basks in the security of knowing that her mother loves her more than anyone else ever could—even more than the government of the United States of America! On the other hand, Harper is uncomfortable with her parents' growing alignment with ultraconservative values and is afraid of the critical perspective and judgmental attitude that seem to be an integral part of their new value system.

Harper the Bookbat

Although Harper is uneasy about a number of her parents' convictions, she is particularly worried about the new, strong position they have taken regarding her reading habits. As Hank and Beth come to view the Bible through a literal, fundamentalist lens, they also come to recognize the authority and power that texts can play in people's lives. Thus, it does not take long before all texts, including Harper's beloved books, become suspect in their eyes. Although Beth is somewhat willing to tolerate Harper's reading interests, Hank fears that his little girl's spiritual life is being threatened by the worldly ideas proliferated in the pages of storybooks. Harper fears that her reading days are numbered and registers immediate concern. She decides then and there that she cannot give up the safe harbor she finds in books, and determines that she will do whatever it takes to ensure that she is able to continue reading, even if it means doing some pretending and being a bit less than honest about her interests and activities.

When a church friend refers to Harper as a "bookworm," she is insulted by the moniker and creates a new identity for herself. In her mind, she declares herself a "bookbat," one who will glide gracefully through any difficult circumstances she encounters, by wisely maneuvering through the world of books. She feels certain that she can continue to please her parents while carving out a new undercover life for herself. Harper realizes that this new identity may require a good bit of surreptitious behavior, but she can see no way around it: "The bookbat in me knew that my books were as important to my survival as food to eat and air to breathe. They helped me navigate. I knew I was doing the right thing. . . . Mom and Dad were so happy. I just wanted them to stay that way and if my being sneaky helped, so what?" (36). Harper's sneakiness did seem to help. When her parents and their church friends took an even stronger position on the inappropriateness of controversial literature, Harper knew just what to do. She turned to one of her favorite literary characters for inspiration and determined that she would outsmart them, Brer Rabbit style. She would continue to read exactly what she wanted, while giving the appearance of growing more and more committed to the church's ideals. Harper's plan worked, and she was able to maintain a relative sense of peace for a while. However, life soon took a turn that she had not expected.

Rolling with the Jessups

The Jessups' church life soon spread beyond the boundaries of the church walls. Just as church had come into their home in the form of visits from well-meaning members, it also extended beyond their borders in the name of missionary involvement. Before long, Harper's parents take up arms in the battle against secular humanism in the schools, becoming outspoken critics of textbooks deemed blasphemous by their church coalition. When Mr. Jessup makes a televised statement along these lines, their life is changed forever. Their church leaders soon declare that the Jessups are no longer mere children of God. Rather, they are called to be His workers—"migrants for God," sent forth to bring truth to the blasphemous public school system.

Before Harper realizes what has happened, the coalition outfits the family with a brand-new Grand Deluxe Roadmaster, a mobile home that is bigger and better than their old one and that will transport them to their new mission field in the heartland of America. Harper discovers that this means she and Weesie will each have her own room and that Harper's room comes equipped with a tiny secret compartment in the floorboards, complete with a lock—a perfect place for hiding her books of choice. She is ecstatic at the Jessups' good fortune but also experiences a sense of dissonance between her spiritual and material values.

Life on the road is difficult for Harper in a number of ways. Although the Jessups' new status within the church coalition brings better living conditions, increased financial security, and, at least for her parents, a sense of prestige and belonging, it also results in the loss of stability. The constant moves take Harper in and out of school systems, making it even more difficult for her to make friends and build solid relationships outside of home. Even when she remains in a particular location for an extended period of time, her parents' strict regulations prevent her from becoming an integral part of the school community.

Time and again, Harper finds herself relegated to the school library, surrounded only by books and, occasionally, a few other students from families with similar viewpoints. Harper does not see this enforced isolation as a hardship, but rather as an opportunity to be alone with her thoughts and to engage in the voracious reading that she loves. She also feels a sense of accomplishment, knowing that in spite of her parents' best efforts to shield her from outside influences and ideas, the Brer Rabbit inside of her has tricked them and won this round of the battle.

All in the Family

In spite of Harper's isolation, there are a number of adults who try to make positive inroads into her life and learning. Caring teachers, insightful school personnel, and interested librarians recognize Harper's intellectual prowess, as well as her emotional longings, and attempt to give her the support she needs in these areas. However, outside of being able to provide Harper with the books she craves, they are able to find few areas of intervention. Adults from beyond the church who do try to break into the Jessups' circle are not received well and run the risk of being labeled as heretics. Thus, many of the people Harper meets learn quickly that they must keep their distance from her parents. When Harper begins to recognize the harsh, mean-spirited, and closed-minded image that surrounds the family's identity, she feels ashamed and desperate.

To make matters more difficult, the Jessups' strife in personal relationships is not limited to mere acquaintances; it extends to family members as well. While on the road, the Jessups take a detour to visit Gammy Beth's mother and Harper and Weesie's grandmother. Harper is delighted to see Gammy—a woman who has exciting ideas, tells thrilling stories, and loves her grandchildren passionately. However, when Gammy crosses the line and tells the girls a story that Hank deems to be ungodly and inappropriate, a battle ensues.

Before the night is out, the Jessups are on the road again, speeding on to the next leg of their missionary journey and leaving the blasphemous Gammy behind. When Beth explains that they are making this move out of a sense of love and conviction, Harper is stunned, confused, and grief stricken. Once again, Harper finds herself cut off from the outside world and caught between her commitment and loyalty to her parents and her desire to have a real life outside of the immediate family and the church cause.

The Gray Zone

When the Jessups' missionary work finally takes them to California, Harper finds a bit of hope. With so much work to be done, it was decided that the Jessups would remain in one locality for an entire year, making it possible for Harper to complete the whole eighth grade without having to change schools even once. To make things even better, the public library is located within easy walking distance of their motor home site. During her very first visit to the library, Harper made a friend.

Harper met Gray Willette in the science fiction section. Their common interests and precocious reading habits made them immediate soul mates. When Harper describes her parents' uneasiness with controversial issues, Gray volunteers to help by hiding Harper's books at his house and invites her to visit anytime she wishes. Gray's home turns out to be different from anything Harper has ever seen before. With family relationships as light and airy as the sunny interior of their house, the Willettes defy every convention Harper has ever known.

As eighth grade progresses, Harper continues to take great pleasure in her books and for the first time, revels in the joys of friendship and the camaraderie that occurs among school-age peers. Yet, even these very positive turns have a downside, in that the sharp contrasts between home and school, and between Gray's world and her own, force Harper to see the problems in her family's life with greater clarity than ever before. Fearing that she will displease her parents, she continues to try to be a model daughter but finds herself hiding between two worlds.

Eventually, however, it becomes impossible to hide the truth that she is no longer the obedient, compliant little girl that her parents want her to be. In spite of her smiles and low-key approach, Harper comes to see home as "alien territory" (176), a place in which she and her parents must coexist, but which could never be considered a safe haven. She recognizes that her parents have evolved into people whom she no longer knows or understands, and she fears that Weesie has become their un-thinking puppet.

The final blow comes when Harper's parents declare that she and Weesie must take part in an antiabortion march. She is stunned that her parents, the very same parents who have never been willing to talk with her about any aspect of pregnancy, are now insistent that she take part in this rather graphic rally that publicly focuses on the end of pregnancy. Although personally opposed to abortion, she does not feel ready to participate in this event and is appalled to see young Weesie forced to take part in a cause that she does not yet understand.

Aware of Harper's pain, Gray declares her forced participation to be child abuse and steps forward with a plan to rescue Harper not only from the rally but also from her parents' control. As the parade begins, Gray appears out of nowhere and supplies Harper with an alibi that allows her to slip away from her parents and with a cross-country bus ticket that will speed her out of her parents' reach and into Gammy's arms. When all is said and done, a more mature 14-year-old Harper is found living with her grandmother, connected with her friend Gray, and buoyed by a court order that ensures at least a temporary separation from her parents' physical control. It's been a long journey.

DIFFERENTIATION OF THE SELF AND THE IMAGO MODEL

Parents and teachers are in the business of what Virginia Satir (1988) calls "peoplemaking." In order to discharge this awesome responsibility effectively, parents and teachers must understand and practice a great many concepts with impeccable intellectual, emotional, and moral honesty. One of the keys to successful parenting and teaching is a sound understanding of child development information and the impact of its application on children. As "implementers" of this information at the middle and secondary school levels, parents and teachers must open their minds to a most fragile time in children's lives—their adolescence.

The transition from childhood to adulthood is the time in children's lives when significant physical, psychological, intellectual, and spiritual changes take place. Adolescence is a time when children begin their journey of discovering who they are vis-à-vis the world and attempt to figure out how they fit into it. This process includes a series of personal and social conflicts that, when resolved, will yield throughout a child's lifetime operative truths, values, interests, personal vision, and drive "towards becoming the person" the child really is (Frankl, 1998).

As caregivers to adolescents, teachers and parents frequently have a difficult time finding the proper balance between ways to remain included in that adolescent's life and ways to provide and be comfortable with sufficient privacy for the adolescent to bloom into a well-adjusted, functional person. Grandparents, other members of the extended family, and friends of the family can also make important contributions to the development of children.

Parents are faced with addressing their own anxiety associated with the separating from their children that permits their children's individuality to emerge properly. Teachers are also faced with determining what their role should be in helping a student fill the gap that exists in that student's world. Sometimes, teachers have the added challenge of having to negotiate their own feelings about wanting to support the child's separation from parents while the parents are actually obstructing progress in this dimension with rigid posturing on issues that inhibits the natural progression of human development. The other side of the coin may also apply. The teacher may be faced with conflicting feelings between unconditional positive regard and a judgmental stance toward a student whose parents' loose morals and lack of boundary setting interfere with the teacher's ability to teach in ways appropriate to the student's chronological age.

The traditional theories of child development, such as Freud's psychosexual stages, Piaget's cognitive stages, Kohlberg's moral stages, and Erikson's psychosocial stages, each offer a unidimensional perspective on the way a person develops and progresses from birth to death. A more comprehensive approach is needed, one that provides a multidimensional perspective of human growth and development.

A relatively new model, imago relationship therapy, can assist us in broadening the way we think about ourselves and those who are in our care. This construct, developed by Harville Hendrix (1988; 1992), incorporates elements of each of the different developmental theories and gives us a new possibility of applying this knowledge. In addition to taking developmental psychology into account, it integrates key elements of the psychotherapeutic models of behavioral, cognitive, psychodynamic, and humanistic psychology. A model that was originally developed to assist couples in deepening the empathic bond between them and in navigating from the "reactive relationship or power struggle" into the "conscious or intentional relationship," it has been augmented to include a model for better caregiving for children (Hendrix and Hunt, 1997).

The imago relationship model for parenting is based on the premise that people who parent successfully create successful relationships in other areas as well, such as marriage or other committed partnerships (Hendrix and Hunt, 1997). The two types of relationships have some basic similarities. Both types of relationships progress through stages. They both begin with the two participants developing an attachment to one another, progress to the emergence of a power struggle, and finally, when the power struggle is successfully managed and directed, culminate in a productive, appropriate, interdependent partnership. The internalized image, or "imago," of one's own caregivers is the catalyst for the interactions that occur in the relationship.

Imago relationship theory postulates that a person's choice for a life partner is affected by the internal image of one's caregivers that is etched in the unconscious. All of these positive and negative interactions become the database from which one makes choices about relationships. The way in which people then nurture their own children is influenced by the internalized experiences they have had with their own caregivers.

To successfully parent or teach children, parents and teachers must become "conscious" of their own imago so that they can use that knowledge to create an intentional relationship, instead of a reactive one, with their children or students. When parents become aware of the behaviors in their child to which they have an intense reaction (either positive or negative), they can begin healing their own childhood wounds and become intentional in their relationships.

In writing about the imago model of parenting, Hendrix and Hunt (1997) make some basic observations about families:

- Wounding gets passed on as a legacy (poor parenting tends to be repeated intergenerationally).
- The place people get stuck in parenting is an indication of where they are stunted psychologically (parents cannot give children that which they have not received themselves).
- Conscious parents must do the same thing that conscious partners do to maintain connection in their relationships (they must change their tendency to react negatively, to criticize, to judge, and to become defensive).

When creating conscious relationships, it is important to keep in mind that the most important difference between a parent-child relationship and a relationship between two adults is that, in the latter, the adults must stretch to meet the needs of each other. In the parent-child relationship, parents must stretch to meet the needs of the child but must have their own needs met within the confines of an adult relationship.

CONSCIOUS PARENTING

Conscious parents are constantly aware of their children's needs and approach meeting those needs with interest and enthusiasm. Among the most basic needs of every child are the need to survive, the need to feel alive, the need to express this aliveness, and the need to maintain a connection to a state of relaxed joyfulness. When the parent excessively restrains or represses the child, wounding occurs. The child's ability to remain relaxed and joyful decreases, and the child experiences a disconnection with the world, especially with the adult in question.

Unconscious parenting is wounding to children. Parents are unconscious when they lack a conscious grasp of their beliefs, actions, behaviors, and feelings. When these things are "out of awareness," they are, therefore, out of control. Many people live in an unconscious state, operating in a way that is akin to automatic pilot, with little self-direction or self-awareness. Because the state of consciousness/unconsciousness exists on a continuum, people's level of consciousness fluctuate over time. (For a full exploration of conscious parenting, see Hendrix and Hunt's 1997 text *Giving the Love That Heals: A Guide for Parents*.)

To fully understand the construct of unconsciousness in the imago model, it is important to understand the role that symbiosis plays in relationships, the character structure of the "missing self," and how developmental wounding causes people to become the people they are, complete with a particular brand of adaptation behaviors for survival. Unconscious relating can be identified best when an interaction cuts the connection between the two people in a relationship. It also disconnects a child from parts of the self that are natural to the child as a human being. This results in children learning that they must shed parts of themselves in order to survive and avoid abandonment, rejection, and shame.

The imago relationship model purports that when children voyage through stages of relational development, wounding is unavoidable because the caregivers come to the table with wounds of their own. If the caregiver has not yet begun the journey into healing, the child will inherit the caregiver's wounds. Additionally, wounding occurs as a matter of life's natural progression because no caregiver can provide a child with every single response necessary to avoid wounding altogether.

As children progress through the developmental stages of life, they tend to adapt to wounding in several ways within two general categories. A child will respond either by becoming a minimizer or by becoming a maximizer. Minimizers are people who tend to constrict or diminish affect. They are independent, withholding, excluding of others, self-centered, compulsive, implosive, and dominant. Maximizers, on the other hand, tend to expand or exaggerate affect. They are dependent, grasping, diffuse, overinclusive of others, other-centered, impulsive, explosive, and submissive (Hendrix and Hunt, 1997).

THE JESSUP FAMILY: LOOKING CLOSELY

Ideally, the goal of any healthy family is to provide a safe, stimulating environment where all members, whether individually or in subsets, have the opportunity to thrive physically, emotionally, intellectually, and spiritually. The ideal environment is a system with components that facilitate open, clear, and direct communication. It should have well-established operational family rules and a clear understanding of each family member's role, responsibilities, and privileges.

The Jessup family system is a closed one. In this family, the members of the system must be cautious about what they say. Harper hides many of her true thoughts when she is in the company of her parents or their friends. Beth experiences a great deal of anxiety when her daughters are asked questions by people from her church because she fears that their responses will not meet the expectations of the people she wants to please. This need to please others through her children, who for her are a reflection of herself, is also illustrative of symbiotic fusion. She shapes her children's behavior so that her need for approval by others is met through the children. She blindly assumes that her children feel the same way she does about "the cause" and the books and issues that they discuss.

The central rule in the Jessup family, as well as in any closed family system, is that everyone is supposed to exhibit the same opinions, feelings, and desires. The rigid rules about who can have membership and enter and exit the system are strictly enforced. Honest self-expression is discouraged because individual and group differences are seen as dangerous to the well-being of the individual and to the survival of family cohesion (Karpel and Strauss, 1983).

The family rules in the Jessup family mandate that Weesie and Harper mold themselves into the same type of religious zealots that their parents are and that the church promotes. Any outside source, such as books (other than the Bible), scientific theories (such as Darwinism), nonmembers of the church (such as Gray, teachers, and librarians), or activities that do not directly reinforce the dogma that will make the children conform to "the right ways," is seen as dangerous by the Jessups. The cause of eradicating the roots of evil in society and schools takes precedence over any rights individuals might have.

The Jessup children are systematically exposed to continual wounding in their family. Harper and Weesie have parents who try to constrict and repress their thoughts, actions, and feelings. They try to encourage those pieces of their children of which they approve and shame those pieces that they do not wish to see. Harper is conscious of the impact her parents' interactions have on her. She is also conscious of the impact that her parents have on her sister. She recognizes that she will not be able to save her sister but that she can help herself by becoming her own caregiver. She uses her courage to embrace and nurture her lost self (her shadow) by surviving emotionally, psychologically, and spiritually.

Collectively, Hank and Beth are inconsistently available to their children because of the self-absorption that results from their lifestyle in the church. For them, the church creates a connection that was missing earlier in their relationship. When they discover a common cause in which they can participate, they suddenly change from being conflictual and abusive to each other, and team up in the pursuit of straightening out the world with religious truths.

As parents, Hank and Beth are overprotective, possessive, and guilty of selectively mirroring their children, while at the same time withholding any information or instructions other than that which is strictly censored. This very wounding type of parenting creates in Harper a child who is confused and scared. She is fighting to acknowledge and experiment with the impulses that are emerging in herself, such as curiosity, the need for knowledge, the need for intellectual stimulation, the need to listen to others' opinions, the need to look at scientific observations, and the need for friends outside of the family circle, while at the same time wrestling with the desire to comply with her parents' wishes. She struggles to have her parents see her as separate and different from them, and she wishes for them to see her as valuable and successful in meeting their standards. She continually holds out the hope that at least her mother will come around and visit her in her world and encourage her to keep growing as she has.

In her attempts to survive, Harper adapts by becoming a minimizer who withholds feelings, is independent, and withdraws into herself. She isolates herself and then manipulates her parents through lies. She tries to champion her sister when she sees Weesie being wounded and victimized by her parents, but Harper soon notices that Weesie is a willing participant and a robotlike conformer in her parents' plan. Harper also adapts by aligning herself with Gray's world and the values and lifestyle of the family system she created and lives in while nurturing her missing self.

Gray is the personification of Harper's missing self. He and his family reflect for Harper those areas that were originally deflected during her development. Gray is the product of a family system that is appropriately open and basically nonwounding. Gray is a child with self-esteem and self-confidence. He is encouraged to explore the world and to take risks. He is encouraged to love deeply and to support his friends. His mother, Colleen, is the model mother and a woman who is not afraid to be different. She is intentional in her relationship with her son and Harper. She listens to their concerns and offers guidance, helping them create their own solutions. She respects and nurtures their individuality.

Harper's surrogate family, created by her to meet her own need for survival in the arid, oppressive environment of the Jessups' household, includes the teacher and librarians who recognize in Harper the wounds caused by her family. They, along with Gray and his family, compensate and complement by helping Harper to discover the information she craves. Harper, the bookbat, is able to survive her parents and their legacies despite their strong pull. She is able to survive by nurturing herself in secrecy until she is able to come out of the shadows.

Sometimes, children have to survive their parents and caregivers by becoming their own parents and by learning how to nurture the child within on their own. Teachers, librarians, social workers, clergy, and friends can help children minimize their woundedness by filling the gaps with the information, caring, and support the children crave and need.

SUGGESTED TREATMENT PLAN AND RECOMMENDATIONS FOR SUPPORT

If Harper were to seek counseling, a number of steps could be taken to support her on the path toward wholeness. However, in a family therapy treatment plan, the entire Jessup family would be considered to be a patient. In family systems therapy, an individual, a couple, or any subsystem of the family is viewed as a piece of a larger puzzle (Minuchen, 1974; Sauber, L'Abate, and Weeks, 1985). Although the family may feel that the problem rests solely with one member, the whole family system may need reworking.

The first step in any counseling relationship is the establishment of a strong bond between therapist and patient. In order to build a sense of trust, a sensitive therapist would simply listen to what Harper wished to share. Children who have coped by hiding and pretending will be very sensitive to "being found out." Thus, it is essential that the defenses children have created be permitted to remain in place until they are ready to shed them. With a sense of trust firmly in place, the therapist would then be ready to help Harper with the following treatment components:

- Assist Harper in continuing and completing the initial stage of differentiating the self. The goal here is to help her create a new way to remain connected to her family and still be able to become the person she wants to be. In this stage Harper might be asked to work through a guided activity in which she is asked to describe the ways she is similar to and different from each parent. It is important for Harper to be able to salvage pieces of her relationship with her parents. It is also essential that she feel secure in the knowledge that her roots have value and have created a strong foundation on which she can build for the rest of her life. When clients are encouraged to cut ties completely, it perpetuates the alienation that they already feel. Ideally, Harper needs to be able to own and celebrate what those roots have given her life. Only then will she be able to accept all of herself as good and lovable.

- Lead Harper in an imago relationship therapy technique known as "parent-child dialogue." This intervention will help her to identify the childhood wound that is creating her pain. In the parent-child dialogue, the therapist serves as the parent to whom the child is speaking. The therapist might include questions such as the following: What's it like to be my child? What's it like to live with me? What's your deepest wound with me? What did you need most from me?

- Help Harper work through the grief of the loss of her dream about the ideal family she wanted in comparison with the type she actually got. The therapist can then help Harper work with any anxiety or depression that might result from this loss and adjustment, and should intervene with plenty of support and validation.

- Help Harper to see that her belief system and her thoughts, not the events in her life, cause her to feel the way she does. Teach her that she can take control of her thoughts. Because our thoughts and expectations create our feelings, she can change the way she reacts to her circumstances.

- Help Harper to clarify her values and beliefs so that she can embrace them at a conscious level. This will help her lead a proactive life and make decisions through thoughts, rather than through simple reactions. Values clarification can occur in therapy by utilizing tools designed for that purpose.

- Help Harper work through the anger and disappointment that are present as a result of her parents' ignoring and overcontrolling her. This work is based on the premise that underneath all anger is hurt and that underneath all hurt is an unmet need. Harper's unmet need is that of the freedom to learn and be herself.

- Assist Harper in reconnecting with her parents in a new way. Invite them to attend joint sessions with their daughters. Teach and coach them to have intentional dialogue with their daughters.

- Help Harper to restructure her relationship with Weesie so as to preserve their bond and be enriched by one another.

- Help Harper to develop a larger social network. Coordinate with her guidance counselor and other helping personnel. Harper might also benefit from group therapy where she is able to share her feelings with other young people who have had similar experiences. This would enable her to "come out" in a safe, protective environment where she can experiment with being the person she has become.

- Assign daily journaling to Harper. Ask her to record all of her thoughts, feelings, and achievements, and coach her on how to communicate these to her parents. Invite Harper to share her journal entries with others in her life, especially the therapist and those in her group therapy network.

Through techniques such as these, a sensitive and competent therapist can play an invaluable role in the lives of children such as Harper. However, many children who are struggling along the road to healthy development never find their way into a formal counseling setting. Therefore, it is also important to consider the significant contributions that concerned parents and teachers can make in helping budding adolescents to develop a positive self-concept, to create a healthy identity separate from their families of origin, and to make steady progress on their journey through the stages of human development.

RECOMMENDED READING

Fiction

Calvert, P. (1989). *When Morning Comes*. New York: Scribner's. 153 pp. (ISBN:0–684–19105–9). HS.

Cat Kincaid is a tough young woman who is living a dangerous life. After being moved through a series of foster homes, she finds herself living with Annie, a kindly beekeeper who understands that Cat's identity runs far deeper than her hard exterior.

Curtis, C. P. (1995). *The Watsons Go to Birmingham—1963*. New York: Scholastic. 210 pp. (ISBN:0–590–69014–0). ES, MS.

Their friends call them the "weird Watsons," but 10-year-old Kenny knows he has a good life, complete with loving parents, an "official juvenile delinquent brother," and an adorable baby sister. What Kenny doesn't know is that his family's trip to Birmingham will lead them to a life-changing moment in the history of the civil rights movement.

Danziger, P., and A. M. Martin. (1998). *P.S. Longer Letter Later: A Novel in Letters*. New York: Scholastic. 234 pp. (ISBN:0–590–21310–5). ES, MS.

Two best friends, as different as night and day, discover that they need each other more than ever when one is forced to move away. This record of their correspondence shows how both girls come to know each other better as they explore their own identities within the framework of their respective families.

Gregory, K. (1998). *Orphan Runaways*. New York: Scholastic. 151 pp. (ISBN:0–590–60366–3). ES, MS.

Two young brothers flee the wretched conditions of a nineteenth-century orphanage, only to find that life on the streets can be a dangerous and harrowing experience. As they search for hope, family, and security, they discover that they must learn to stand up for what is right.

Holman, F. (1974). *Slake's Limbo*. New York: Aladdin. 117 pp. (ISBN: 0–689–71066–6). MS, HS.

Aremis Slake had led a short and miserable life until, at the age of 13, he could take no more. So, he simply went underground, taking up residence in the New York subway system. In this story of pain, disillusionment, and, ultimately, hope, Slake finds the courage to move into the light of day.

Kerr, M. E. (1972). *Dinky Hocker Shoots Smack*. New York: Dell. 190 pp. (ISBN:0–440–92030–2). MS, HS.

Dinky's parents are so busy solving the problems of the world that they fail to notice the emotional pain that their daughter is experiencing. Dinky finally takes bold steps to make her pain known and to proclaim a personal identity that stands apart from her family's expectations.

Lyons, M. D. (1992). *Letters from a Slave Girl: The Story of Harriet Jacobs*. New York: Simon & Schuster. 175 pp. (ISBN:0–689–80015–0). MS.

Based on a true story, these letters depict Harriet Jacobs's struggles as a young slave. Hurt, afraid, and alone, Harriet must make hard decisions and take serious risks in her pursuit of freedom and a new life.

Oughton, J. (1995). *Music from a Place Called Half Moon*. New York: Houghton Mifflin. 162 pp. (ISBN:0–395–70737–4). MS, HS.

During the summer of 1956, concerns about integration swirled through the Deep South. As 13-year-old Edie Jo sorts through her own passions and prejudices, she discovers that her belief system is shaped one relationship at a time.

Paulsen, G. (1993). *Nightjohn*. New York: Bantam. 92 pp. (ISBN:0–440–21936–1). ES, MS.

A young slave girl longs to learn how to read and write. When her loved ones are forced to pay a painful price for her becoming literate, she must make difficult, adult choices that will affect the future course of her life.

Rylant, C. (1986). *A Fine White Dust*. New York: Dell. 106 pp. (ISBN: 0–440–4299–2). ES, MS.

When Peter met the preacher, he knew that his life would never be the same. Drawn to the man as much as the message, Peter is willing to forsake his family life in order to follow the preacher's vision. This is the story of a young man's evolution into a new adult identity and re-connection with his childhood values.

Nonfiction

Branden, N. (1995). *The Six Pillars of Self-Esteem*. New York: Bantam. 341 pp. (ISBN:0–553–37439–7). HS, A.

A book to help make the connection between psychological problems and low self-esteem.

Faber, A., and E. Mazliash. (1991). *How to Talk So Kids Will Listen and How to Listen So Kids Will Talk*. New York: Avon. 242 pp. (ISBN: 0–380–57000–9). A.

This program teaches the skills necessary to achieve better cooperation from children through communication instead of punishment.

Forward, S., with C. Buck. (1990). *Toxic Parents: Overcoming Their Hurtful Legacy and Reclaiming Your Life*. New York: Bantam. 325 pp. (ISBN:0–553–28434–7). HS, A.

A self-help guide that helps one ask and answer the questions, Am I the child of toxic parents? and, Am I a toxic parent?

Hendrix, H. (1990). *Getting the Love You Want: A Guide for Couples*. New York: Harper Perrenial. 256 pp. (ISBN:0–060–97292–0). A.

This text provides a good introduction to the imago model and provides specific help for couples.

Hendrix, H. (1992). *Keeping the Love You Find: A Guide for Singles*. New York: Simon & Schuster. 327 pp. (ISBN:0–671–73420–2). A.

Based on the imago model, this guide is for singles who desire to be part of a long and loving relationship.

Hendrix, H., and H. Hunt. (1997). *Giving the Love That Heals: A Guide for Parents*. New York: Pocket. 368 pp. (ISBN:0–671–79398–5). A.

This guide applies the imago model and provides valuable information about the ways in which one can be a conscious parent.

REFERENCES

Bowen, M. (1985). *Family Therapy in Clinical Practice*. Northvale, NJ: Jason Aronson.

Clinton, H. R. (1996). *It Takes a Village to Raise a Child, and Other Lessons Children Teach Us*. New York: Simon & Schuster.

Frankl, V. (1998). *Man's Search for Meaning*. New York: Washington Square.

Gurman, A. S., and D. P. Kniskern. (1981). *Handbook of Family Therapy*. New York: Brunner/Mazel.

Hendrix, H. (1988). *Getting the Love You Want: A Guide for Couples*. New York: Harper & Row.

Hendrix, H. (1992). *Keeping the Love You Find: A Guide for Singles*. New York: Simon & Schuster.

Hendrix, H., and H. Hunt. (1997). *Giving the Love That Heals: A Guide for Parents*. New York: Pocket.

Karpel, M., and E. Strauss. (1983). *Family Evaluation*. New York: Gardner.

Lasky, K. (1994). *Memoirs of a Bookbat*. San Diego: Harcourt Brace.

Love, P., and J. Robinson. (1990). *The Emotional Incest Syndrome: What to Do When a Parent's Love Rules Your Life*. New York: Bantam.

Minuchen, S. (1974). *Families and Family Therapy*. Cambridge, MA: Harvard University Press.

Minuchen, S., and H. C. Fishman. (1981). *Family Therapy Techniques*. Cambridge, MA: Harvard University Press.

Satir, V. (1988). *The New Peoplemaking*. Mountain View, CA: Science and Behavioral.

Sauber, R. S., L. L'Abate, and G. R. Weeks. (1985). *Family Therapy: Basic Concepts and Terms*. Baltimore, MD: Aspen Systems.

CHAPTER 6

Identity within the Father-Son Relationship: Robert Newton Peck's *A Day No Pigs Would Die*

Charles R. Duke and Jon L. Winek

INTRODUCTION

Father-son relationships have been the subject of literature from ancient times to the present: Odysseus and his son, Telemachus, in the *Odyssey*, Hamlet and the ghost of his father in Shakespeare's play, Robert and his father in *A Day No Pigs Would Die*. Inherent in all of these relationships is the basic struggle of the son seeking to secure the approval of the father figure while also exerting a sense of independence and identity that permits the son to take his own place in the world and chart his own direction. Not surprisingly, these struggles, in literature as well as in life, are fraught with conflicts ranging from physical confrontation to more subtle yet equally powerful psychological dilemmas. Accompanying such struggles are society's expectations about what constitutes manly attributes and what the best ways may be to live out one's role as a male.

The belief that "as the twig is bent, so grows the tree" places tremendous responsibility on the father figure. From the father, the son has to learn the brutal lessons of masculinity while balancing these lessons against the need for emotional security and a sense of place in the world. The latter two are often supplied by the matriarchal side of the family. Being caught between the male and female sides of parenting presents still another challenge to the young male.

Robert Newton Peck's semiautobiographical novel *A Day No Pigs*

Would Die provides a story about a Vermont Shaker farm boy named Robert, his relationship with his father, Haven Peck, the world as Robert discovers it in Vermont, and his very short journey from childhood to manhood. While the novel may appear to be a simple, nostalgic look at the author's boyhood, the story addresses some basic lessons that, in the author's eyes at least, are best learned from nature and from the "plain" people in one's life.

The novel tracks one year in Robert's life, a year in which he saves a neighbor's cow, raises a prize pig, gets to sample city life, and learns about the values of life and death from both the animal and the human perspectives. In this short span of time, Robert is under constant pressure to learn many life lessons. When his father Haven dies Robert is left to assume the position of head of the household for his mother, aunt, and the farm his father left.

Among the universal questions that the novel presents are the following: (1) How does a son establish his own identity independent of a strong father image? (2) How can a son hope to meet his father's high expectations? (3) How does a son balance the strong male presence of the father against the needs and expectations of a less demanding mother? (4) How does religion play a role in shaping one's sense of self and the world? (5) How does one reconcile the brutality of masculinity with the need for emotion and a sense of place in the world?

SYNOPSIS

From the very beginning of the novel, we sense the ongoing struggle Robert will have in deciding about his own identity. He's not comfortable in dealing with some challenges in a world that has yet to yield to him all its rules of conduct, but when presented with a challenge in his own world, that of nature and the farm, he shows no hesitation in making decisions. For instance, after being bullied by one of his classmates, Robert plays hooky for the rest of the day and retreats to the hills around his father's farm. While there, he sees a cow in distress that is trying to give birth to a calf. At this point Robert thinks, "I'd just wound up running away from Edward Thatcher and running away from the school-house. I was feathered if I was going to run away from one darn more thing" (5). And so he takes action and at considerable risk to himself, assists the cow in giving birth to the calf. Much of his fear and frustration about not knowing exactly what to do comes out in a rather severe and primitive response: "I never hit anybody, boy or beast, as I hit that cow.

I beat her so hard I was crying. Where I held the big cane, the thorns were chewing up my hands real bad. But it only got me madder" (6).

There is always a lesson to be learned in each part of Robert's life. The birth of the calf is important to the continued livelihood of those who make their living from the earth, but there is also a balance to be learned. Robert learns one of many lessons about this balance, which are taught to him by his father in both direct and indirect ways. As Robert is recuperating from his struggle with the cow, he and his father talk. Haven Peck is not one to provide direct praise to anyone, but he can put that praise into a natural context that lets Robert know his father is proud of him while also disappointed that Robert was not consistent in his behavior.

The lessons that Robert is asked to learn with his father's help are not easy ones. They are basic to survival—harsh, direct, and painful. The lessons come quickly during Robert's thirteenth year, helping him, even though he is unaware of it at the time, to be prepared for the time when his father finally dies. Robert learns rapidly just how brutal a man's life can be and that at times such brutality may not be necessary, even if it exists as a part of the masculine code. Such a lesson emerges when he, his father, and a neighbor try to "weasel a dog," a rite of passage for hunting dogs in the area. This practice involves putting a young dog and a weasel in a barrel with a top on it and letting them fight it out until one or the other is dead. In this particular instance, the battle has no victors. The weasel is killed, but Hussy, the dog, emerges from the fight mangled and barely alive.

> "She's dying," I said. "And if you got any mercy at all in you, Ira Long, you'll do her in." . . .
> "Mind your tongue, boy. You're talking to your elders," said Ira.
> "The boy's right," Papa said. "I'll get a gun." (110)

The dog is put out of her misery, and her burial falls to Robert. As he places her in the ground, he says, "Hussy . . . you got more spunk in you than a lot of us menfolk got brains" (111).

Father and son have great difficulty showing how strong the emotional ties are between them. Haven Peck is not given to many words in dealing with his family, and when he does speak, it is almost always in the form of some kind of teaching. But father and son come to know that the bond that holds them together runs deep and true, especially as Haven, who knows he is dying, tries to prepare his son for life without him.

The creation of an emotional bond between father and son culminates in the killing of Pinky, Robert's one prized possession. Robert was given the pig by a neighbor as a reward for saving the neighbor's calf. Robert raises the pig only to discover that she is barren and can provide no ongoing supply of meat. In the adult world, as Haven has tried to teach his son, everything must have a purpose. Without Pinky's fertility, there will be no continuing source of meat, and the cost of feeding the barren pig is too high to sustain. "That's what being a man is all about, boy. It's just doing what's got to be done" (139). Father and son, therefore, share in the killing of Pinky, and it is in that culminating moment that both father and son acknowledge, again without words, their love and understanding of each other.

Robert has other lessons to learn about growing up. Some of these come from the female side of the family and focus more on education and appearance. Haven Peck's wife and her sister, Carrie, offer the maternal side to Robert's development. They are seen primarily as shadowy figures, ones who emphasize the importance of education—something that Haven's father also preaches—and who tend to the sick and who look to the male figures in their lives to take care of the more demanding and unpleasant aspects of life. Robert is so caught up in trying to work out his relationship with his father that he fails, until just before his father's death, to see that his role as a man encompasses more than just tilling the land and taking care of the livestock. As his father tells him, "It can't be no longer your mother and Carrie taking care of you. Soon you got to care for them. They're old too. Years of work done that" (122).

One of the influences that permeate Robert's growth into manhood are the simple, direct, and unwavering religious beliefs of the Shakers. Although neither Haven Peck nor his wife can read or write, they find a way to translate the basic Shaker beliefs into a code of conduct and life, which they transmit to Robert more through actions than words. As a result of these beliefs, Robert knows that he and his family are different from the Baptists who also live in the area. Accepting those differences is difficult for Robert at first, but he slowly comes to realize that his neighbors, most of whom are Baptists, have a strong admiration for his father and how he lives. Time and again, the Shaker beliefs focus Robert's attention on what is acceptable. For example, he desperately wants a bicycle like the other children in the village, but he knows his chances of getting one are slim. Another time, Robert tells his father he needs a new store-bought coat for winter. His father tells him that needs aren't important but deeds are.

The life of Robert Peck is not an easy one. His "time in training" to become a man is short and, for the most part, rough. Most of his lessons are learned through direct experience, and most of them come from his father. Confronted as he is with the realities of the plain, simple life his father and mother live, in which there is little time for reflection and in which emotion is only hinted and never expressed, Robert has to figure out his own role as reflected through the actions of others.

The Shaker way of life leaves little room for a young man to reflect on lessons learned or those yet to come. Such a life places tremendous pressure on the individual growing up. In a world where direct expression of affection or acceptance between father and son is rare, where finding oneself in the minority as an adolescent offers social adjustment problems, and where females are placed in subordinate roles, the adolescent male can be expected to be looking for help, understanding, and answers.

THERAPY WITH ROBERT

Systemic family therapy is an approach to working with clients that recognizes the natural context within which clients function. Adolescence is a period of rapid personal and physical growth. Given this, it is expected to be a difficult period of transition for all members of a family. A youth having difficulty in this period of life is a good candidate for family therapy. In fact, many problems adults face in terms of their relationships have origins that are traceable to difficulties in their adolescent years. For instance, adult problems with addictions and intimacy often have origins in difficulties during adolescence. So, as a therapist, it is far better to try to help adolescents with issues before they enter adulthood. If the issues are not addressed until adulthood, they become more fixed. The extreme flux that an adolescent personality undergoes is what makes working with adolescents most rewarding and most challenging.

Given the simple Shaker ways of Robert's parents, it is unlikely that they would be willing to come with Robert for family therapy. This would not matter since systems therapists are well equipped to deal with individuals as they struggle with family issues and would be very comfortable, and capable of, working with Robert individually.

While his Shaker life leaves little room for Robert to reflect on the lessons that life has tried to teach, this is just what a therapist would strive to do with young Robert. In working with Robert, it would be important to work within his faith. While one might view his family's faith as something that hinders his development, this is not necessarily the case. An alternative, and ultimately more useful, view of it would be to see his faith as a source of support for this young man. Robert's faith provides him with a clear sense of right and wrong and a strong sense of community.

In families that have a strong sense of independence and pride in that independence, it is unlikely that they would seek out a therapist. More often, a referral would come from the school. Robert's difficulties at school are implied in the very beginning of the book, where he talks of being made fun of by other children and of getting revenge. He states that this revenge will be in the form of physical violence.

Robert does not like school and is doing poorly. This is typical, considering the stress Robert is under at home. Children who are under severe stress often act out in the system that is less stressful. Robert is struggling to develop into a man. He is also struggling with his relationship with his parents, especially his father. In a very real way, he is being forced to deal with life-and-death issues at an early age. With all of these stressors operating in his home life, one would expect that Robert would have problems in school. Further, these problems would come to the attention of the school counselor or a concerned teacher, so it is likely that the school would refer him for therapy.

The first goal of therapy would be to develop a relationship of trust with Robert. Most likely, at first Robert would have a hard time talking to a therapist. Not knowing the therapist, he would speak in the most formal, respectful, and reserved manner that he could muster. At one point, when thinking about asking his neighbor a question, Robert thinks, "But I remembered my 'manners' and owed up to silence. 'Never miss a chance,' Papa had once said, 'to keep your mouth shut.' And the more I studied on it, the sounder it grew" (91).

In addition, he would not be experienced at talking about his emotions. In his family, emotions are a luxury and best left to the women. However, over time a relationship could be developed as a result of the therapist's actively seeking to develop such a relationship with him. Robert would eventually feel free to speak without censorship about what he was thinking and feeling. The best way to encourage Robert to speak freely would be to model such behavior. By sharing thoughts and speaking about things that matter, the therapist would gain Robert's trust.

At first, whatever Robert brought to the therapy session would be accepted without judgment. The therapist would simply listen, for example, as he described his relationships with the important characters in his life. While active listening seems such a simple task, in fact, listening well is one of the most difficult skills that a counselor must learn. It's very easy to get caught up in the story and share one's feelings about what is going on without even knowing it. However, the therapist's sharing reflections on the lessons in Robert's life is of little use. But by talking about and reflecting on the lessons that his own life is offering, Robert can grow as an individual.

While a therapist's goal would be to encourage Robert to speak freely, the therapist would need to consider Robert's developmental level. Rarely does a teen speak freely to an adult. Given this, the therapist's active listening would need to be more intense than it would need to be with an adult. For example, when asked an open question, the most common response a teen will give is "I don't know." However, this statement can have several meanings. Most commonly, it means "I am not comfortable telling you that." Unless the therapist probes and asks slightly leading questions, the adolescent client can shut down and not communicate.

For example, if Robert shared the story of weaseling the dog (105–111) in a therapy session, it would be hard for the therapist not to pass judgment on this practice. However, careful selection of questions would lead to exploration of important issues without being evaluative. The following dialogue, with Dr. Winek in the therapist's role, is an example of how the interview might go:

Dr. Winek: So why was the dog put in a barrel with a weasel?

Robert: It's to make Hussy hate the weasel.

Dr. Winek: So why does a dog need to hate a weasel?

Robert: So they will know to keep them out of the henhouse.

Dr. Winek: I see—so your dad and Ira were trying to teach Hussy her nature.

Robert: Right.

Dr. Winek: But it did not work; it only resulted in both dog and weasel being killed.

Robert: Yeah, so I guess Hussy didn't learn about her nature.

Dr. Winek: I think Hussy learned about her nature, but the cost was too high. Learning about your nature at the cost of your life is not a good lesson. But what about the dog's other nature? You know, the sweet nature that you felt when she sat in your arms all the way home. Was that part of Hussy's nature that you men could have been taught about by the dog, rather than trying to teach the dog to be a killer?

Robert: Yeah, I guess we could have learned that from Hussy.

Dr. Winek: How did all of this make you feel?

Robert: I don't know.

Dr. Winek: Sure you do. Often when some experience is very intense like this, your emotions get all mixed together. It helps if you just name them and sort them out after you name them.

Robert: I guess I felt mad, sad, and embarrassed.

Dr. Winek: Good, let's look at your anger first. What were you mad about?

Robert: I was angry that such a sweet dog got killed. I was angry at that weasel. But that's just his nature, except in nature you don't find yourself in a barrel with a dog. I guess I was also angry at my father for catching the weasel.

Dr. Winek: Are you still mad at your dad?

Robert: Not really. Even though he didn't say it, he was very sorry. I know he did not mean for anything bad to happen.

Dr. Winek: What about your sorrow?

Robert: Mostly for Hussy. But, you know, I feel a little sorrow for the weasel.

Dr. Winek: Like you said, it is not his nature to fight a dog in a barrel.

Robert: Exactly.

Dr. Winek: I think it was good that you had to bury Hussy. That gave you a little time with your sorrow. It's not like you wanted to bury her, but it was probably good for you to have a little bit of time alone. You know, to say good-bye. It's important to spend time with and express our grief. It's part of our nature to feel grief when we experience a loss.

Robert: I guess you're right. I said my good-byes. I guess even people got nature.

Dr. Winek: That's very true. The tragedy is that few people ever find their nature. I guess that even fewer yet look for it.

Robert: Seems like my nature is finding me.

Dr. Winek: That seems about right. What about your embarrassment?

Robert: Things turned out so bad I felt like a damn fool for taking part in such a mess.

Dr. Winek: Do you think the others felt that way, too?

Robert: They didn't say as much, but I reckon that would be true.

An exchange such as the one described above between Robert and his therapist would allow Robert a rare opportunity to reflect on the emotional impact of this dramatic event in his life. Few parents and even fewer fathers invite their children to focus on the emotional ramifications of their experiences. Like the act of placing a young dog in a barrel with a weasel, the lessons of masculinity are often brutal. This brutality can stem not only from action but also from the repression of strong emotions, like anger, sadness, and embarrassment. By tempering the lessons of masculinity with the real expression of emotions, a young man can be given the opportunity to develop emotional security and a sense of place in the world. Such a conversation also helps the son to develop an identity that transcends the image he has of his father.

DR. WINEK'S RECOMMENDATIONS

If I were Robert's therapist, I would not criticize the father or seek to alter the boy's image of his father. Rather I would simply seek to build on Robert's image of his father. Sons naturally strive to imitate their fathers' identities. By adding to this natural developmental process the ability to process and accept his own emotional experience, Robert can develop his own independent identity. Since this new identity does not require rejection of the image of the father, but simply builds upon it, the chances for intergenerational conflict (and, ultimately, rejection of the son by the father) are greatly reduced. If Robert were encouraged to question and reject portions of his father, there would likely be an emotional and, quite possibly a real, cutoff of relations between the generations.

It is easy to think that all of Robert's issues in therapy would be with his father, but Robert will need to find a balance between his father's strong presence and the expectations of a less demanding mother. In unhealthy families this tension can get resolved by the mother intervening in the relationship between father and son. This can be referred to as "triangulation"—the boy becomes closer to his mother than the father is to his wife, setting up a destructive competition between father and son that in extreme cases gets resolved by the dissolution of the marital relationship. If I sensed Robert's mother becoming overinvolved, I would try to disrupt this pattern. However, in Peck's book, it is clear that the mother takes an appropriate supportive role. She seems comfortable in her relationship to both of the men in her life, caring for both in separate ways that do not put the men in competition for her attentions. This is one of the factors that make me optimistic for a favorable resolution to this difficult period in Robert's life.

Robert's father has such high expectations that Robert must struggle to meet them. There is a strong emotional connection between father and son. However, the father has a limited way of expressing his feelings toward his son. By always providing his son a lesson in life, Robert's father expresses his care for his son, a common pattern among men as they try to rear their male children. Men typically express care through actions. By teaching the male child the tasks that are associated with manhood, the father feels a strong connection to his son. I would expect that Robert's father had a similar relationship to his father as he was growing up.

This style of relating is not as unique to Robert's family as one might think. Nor is it unique to families with strong religious beliefs like the Shakers. A young boy's struggle to live up to his father's ideal must be resolved by many men. While the style of relating seen between Robert and his father is common, there are some shortfalls to this practice. First, the caring often becomes expressed as a set of expectations, and this set of expectations can become a burden for the child unable to meet them. The father may at this point reach out for his son. However, this takes the form of more lessons and more expectations. Thus a common but tragic family pattern is established. The father becomes critical in order to encourage his son. The son fails out of anxiety, resulting in further criticism from the father. This can then become a vicious cycle that is very difficult for each to resolve.

This pattern can be broken by having the father and son learn to express their shared connection in ways other than lessons and expectations. In Robert's case this issue becomes more critical. Robert's father is in touch with the fact that his own health is a serious issue. When his father shares this awareness, Robert longs for a touch, a kiss, or more discussion. Instead his father just goes to bed (122).

After hearing about this in therapy, it would be important to help Robert face the emotional issues between himself and his father. I would encourage Robert to share *his feelings* with his father. If Robert just waits for his father to reach out to him, it is not likely to happen. Robert is in touch with his feelings. However, my concern is that if they do not get expressed, his feelings will become repressed, and often such repressed feelings get played out in future relationships. Most likely, in Robert's case this would get played out with his own son.

Since Robert is in touch with his feelings, the first step would be to encourage him to express his feelings toward his father in the safety of the therapy session. After he was more comfortable expressing these feelings in therapy, I would encourage Robert to share how he feels with his father.

There would be some risk that his father might not be able to hear Robert's expression. I would point out to Robert that the power of expressing love is not in the receiving, but in the giving. Once Robert appreciates this, he is in a win-win situation. Even if his father does not acknowledge Robert's expression of love, Robert would still benefit.

Father and son are able to acknowledge their love and understanding without words as they share in the killing of Pinky. The difference that therapy could make in Robert's life is that successful therapy would allow for the addition of expressing this love with words. Given his history, this would be a different goal indeed. It would most likely take some pushing for Robert to draw on the strength of the therapist-client relationship. Here I would break my rule against providing the client with advice. I would want to advise Robert to discuss his relationship with his father before it was too late. That session in which I push Robert to discuss his feelings might go something like this:

Dr. Winek: Sounds like a very powerful experience occurred between yourself and your father when you had to butcher Pinky.

Robert: Yes. It was the hardest thing I ever had to do. I realize that we were just doing what we had to, but it was still hard. When he looked away from me and wiped the tears, I knew he had strong feelings like me. I knew he loved Pinky, and I knew he loved me.

Dr. Winek: That's great. A lot of boys never know that their dads love them. I know this will be hard to hear, but as you discussed before, your father is not well. In fact he thinks he will be dying soon.

Robert: [Starting to cry] I know, and I don't want him to die.

Dr. Winek: I know that. You do love your father. That's why it is going to be important for you to find the words to tell him that.

Robert: Don't you think he knows? Like I know he loves me.

Dr. Winek: Yes, but it is also important to speak this directly. I have worked with a lot of men who have lost their fathers. They are troubled because they think of things they would like to tell their fathers, but they feel it's too late. It's very hard, but it's not too late for you. You needed to say good-bye to Hussy and Pinky. You're going to need to say good-bye to your father, and it's important that you do it while he is still alive. That way he can say good-bye to you.

Robert: [Crying] I know, but I just don't know what to say.

Dr. Winek: [Long pause letting Robert cry] I know. That's what we can work on here.

I would hope some of the grief work that Robert will have to do can be done prior to his father's death. But even if so, there will still be much to be done afterward. Robert's therapy would continue for at least a year but more likely would continue for closer to two years. In the therapy I would continue to support Robert's struggle to become a man. After the death of his father, the relationship between Robert and myself would likely shift. Robert probably would transfer some of the feelings he had toward his father to me. It would be important to recognize this and not allow myself to forget that I am not his father. I would want to be supportive but not allow Robert to become dependent on me. This is a difficult balance to find, but one that must be found in almost all therapeutic relationships.

While Robert's Shaker life favors the father-son relationship, their struggle is both ancient and universal. All sons and fathers have to work on their relationships as the sons grow. In particular, they have to resolve several dichotomies. Specifically, the balance between masculinity and femininity; pride and disappointment; courage and fear. Furthermore, sons need to decide whether to adopt their fathers' values and beliefs. Regardless of how these dilemmas are resolved, sons and fathers will pay an emotional and relational price. Therapy can reduce this price by allowing the participants to examine and choose their actions more carefully. During this process, clients are inclined to believe their struggles are unique to them. By reading and talking about others who struggle with similar dilemmas, clients often can discover options that were previously invisible. Discovering the options that lie between the two extremes often means that a father and son can forge a more meaningful relationship.

RECOMMENDED READINGS

Fiction

Bauer, Marion Dare. (1993). *Face to Face*. New York: Dell. 192 pp. (ISBN: 0–440–40791–5). MS.

Eight years after he has abandoned his family, Bret invites his son, Michael, to go white-water rafting in Colorado. The river trip shows Michael what a bully his father is and helps Michael come to understand that Dave, his stepfather, loves him just the way he is—Michael does not have to change to be accepted.

Brown, James. (1994). *Lucky Town*. New York: Harcourt Brace. 287 pp. (ISBN: 0–15–100067–0). HS.

In this coming-of-age novel, Bobby Barlow recalls his teen years, when he lived a lawless life with his ex-convict father, and the influence these years had on Bobby's later life.

Buchanan, William J. (1992). *One Last Time*. New York: Avon Flare. 118 pp. (ISBN: 0–380–76152–1). MS, HS.

Young David Baca, part Apache, part Isleta, becomes a vaquero to help his father with range work. When a maverick bull gores his father, David accepts the challenge of ridding the range of the bull and making the range safe for all.

Close, Jessie. (1990). *The Warping of Al*. New York: HarperCollins. 282 pp. (ISBN: 0–060–21280–2). HS.

Al tries to live up to his father's expectations but finds it impossible since Al wants to be a chef and his father wants him to go into a regular business.

Crutcher, Chris. (1995). *Ironman*. New York: Greenwillow. 140 pp. (ISBN: 0–688–13503–X). MS, HS.

Beauregard Brewster is constantly in trouble at school. He eventually discovers that much of his hostility and pain is rooted in his relationship with his father and that running in a triathlon will not solve the problem.

Davis, Ossie. (1992). *Just Like Martin*. New York: Simon & Schuster. 215 pp. (ISBN: 0–671–73202–1). MS.

Stone meets Dr. Martin Luther King Jr. in 1963 in Alabama and wants to grow up to be just like him. Stone's father, an embittered Korean War veteran, despises nonviolence and refuses to accept it as a way of life. Stone becomes caught between his love for his father, who carries a gun in his pickup at all times, and Stone's own emerging beliefs and values.

DeClements, Barthe. (1990). *Monkey See, Monkey Do*. New York: Delacorte. 146 pp. (ISBN: 0–385–30158–8). MS.

When Jerry's father is released from prison, Jerry's greatest hope is that his father will stay clean and not have to go back. In spite of the best efforts of Jerry and his mother, Jerry Sr. breaks his parole and is arrested again, leaving Jerry to struggle with adjusting to life without him once again.

Delffs, Dudley J. (1993). *Forging August*. New York: Pinion. 257 pp. (ISBN: 0–89109–747–3). MS, HS.

This novel develops the story of 18-year-old Bounty, who is the pawn in his parents' divorce. We witness the father's authoritarian attitude and the mother's dependency played out against the politics of a small Tennessee town and see how Bounty has to negotiate his way to finding his own identity.

Ferris, Jean. (1996). *All That Glitters*. New York: Farrar, Straus & Giroux. 184 pp. (ISBN: 0–374–30204–9). MS, HS.

Brian gets to spend six weeks in the Florida Keys with his father, from whom he is estranged. Brian wishes for a father more like that of Nathan, his neighborhood friend. The six weeks Brian spends with his father, however, enable him to come to a better understanding of their relationship, especially after going through a hurricane with him.

Halecroft, David. (1990). *Breaking Loose*. New York: Viking. 114 pp. (ISBN: 0–670–84697–X). MS, HS.

Matt Greene is one of the best football players the Alden Panthers have ever seen, and he seems destined to be a star. But his dad, a former NFL All-Pro, wants Matt to become an instant star. Trying to live up to his father's expectations, Matt starts fumbling, missing plays, and causing everyone, including himself, to wonder if he has what it takes.

Nonfiction

Eyre, Richard, and Linda Eyre. (1994). *Three Steps to a Strong Family*. New York: Simon & Schuster. 235 pp. (ISBN: 0–671–88728–9). HS.

The Eyres offer a practical approach to raising responsible children and ensuring that family life brings about a sense of unity. Useful hands-on exercises are included.

Faber, Adele, and Elaine Mazlish. (1982). *How to Talk So Kids Will Listen and Listen So Kids Will Talk*. New York: Avon. 242 pp. (ISBN: 0–380–57000–9). HS.

The authors, drawing upon the work of Dr. Haim Ginott, provide unique suggestions on how to listen to and understand the concerns of children, how to foster cooperation within the family unit, and how to encourage children's development of a positive self-concept.

Fenwick, Elizabeth, and Tony Smith. (1996). *Adolescence: The Survival Guide for Parents and Teenagers*. New York: DK Publishing. 285 pp. (ISBN: 0–7894–0635–7). HS.

The authors divide their comments into four sections: "The Milestones of Adolescence" "Learning to Live Together," "The Adolescent and the Outside World," and "The Adolescent in Trouble." The authors provide both adolescents and parents with useful information about how to travel successfully through the turbulence of growing up.

Rodriguez, Richard. (1993). *Days of Obligation: An Argument with My Mexican Father*. New York: Penguin. 330 pp. (ISBN: 0–670–81396–6). HS.

In this collection of autobiographical essays, Rodriguez explores his own cultural identity and how it has been shaped by his father. Son of an immigrant from Mexico, Rodriguez is a native Californian, but his complexion and features clearly show his Mexican ancestry. He feels keenly the tug of two cultures within him and knows that he must answer to both.

Rosemond, John K. (1996). *Parent Power: A Common-Sense Approach to Parenting in the 90s and Beyond.* Kansas City, MO: Universal Press Syndicate. 231 pp. (ISBN: 0–8362–2808–1). HS.

Rosemond has authored a series on parenting. This third volume focuses on the stages of a child's development and how parents can anticipate the problems that may emerge during each stage. Problem-solving advice is included.

Zumwalt, Elmo, Jr., and Elmo Zumwalt III. (1986). *My Father, My Son.* New York: Macmillan. 224 pp. (ISBN: 0–026–33630–8). HS.

Lieutenant Elmo Zumwalt III was a Navy veteran who became sick with cancer after an exposure to Agent Orange in Vietnam. His father, Admiral Elmo Zumwalt Jr., gave the order that led to the spraying of the defoliant. This joint autobiography traces their journey to the forging of a deep relationship that enabled them to deal with the ordeal.

REFERENCES

Bronfenbrenner, Urie. (1976). "Alienation and the Four Worlds of Childhood." *Phi Delta Kappa* 76 (6): 430–437.

Kaywell, Joan F. (1994). "Using YA Problem Fiction and Non-fiction to Produce Critical Readers." *ALAN Review* 21 (winter): 29–32.

Peck, Robert Newton. (1972). *A Day No Pigs Would Die.* New York: Knopf.

Robson, B. (1993). "Changing Family Patterns: Developmental Impacts on Children." In J. Carlson and J. Lewis (Eds.), *Counseling the Adolescent: Individual, Family and School Improvements*, 2nd ed., Denver, CO: Love, 149–165.

CHAPTER 7

Identity within Societal Expectations: S. E. Hinton's *The Outsiders*

Mary E. Little and Mary Alice Meyers

> Students will not care how much you know until they know how much you care.
>
> —Anonymous

At the heart of the American dream is the belief that all can achieve a life of success, contentment, and fulfillment. It is through the opportunities provided by our society that each and every person realizes individual potential as successful, contributing members within a democratic society. To address the needs of our youngest citizens, various agencies and societal systems have been instituted by the adults within our society. Whether through the family, schools, the judicial system, organized religion, or the community itself, adults are charged with the development, direction, and mentorship of the children. But are the needs of the children being addressed? Have positive changes been occurring for our children and adolescents? The roles and responsibilities of adults and the social services created by adults to address the needs of young people must be reconceptualized because those needs are changing.

The focus of this chapter is to challenge the thinking of adults in light of their roles and responsibilities to children and adolescents, given current research on existing needs and programs, and the efficacy of the basic societal institutions. To personalize the discussions, the novel *The Outsiders*, by S. E. Hinton, was selected. Written initially in 1973 when the author herself was only 16 years of age, this novel was selected because of its timeless appeal to young adults and adolescents.

SYNOPSIS

Following the tragic death of both of his parents, Ponyboy, through whose eyes the story is told, is left to be raised by his two older brothers. While Ponyboy is, by his own admission, a good student who loves to read and who stars on the track team, his teenage brothers, Soda and Darry, are high school dropouts. As brothers, they do not have much in common, except their loyalty to each other. Beyond this brotherly tie, the three teenagers share a bond in that they are members of a street gang called the Greasers.

The Greasers are the low-income ne'er-do-well gang in this anonymous American town. Their chief rivals are the Socs, who are the well-to-do society boys in the same community. Given the social dichotomy, the Greasers feel that they are rejected by their peers outside of their gang; the financial disparities are obvious.

Ponyboy, at 14, is the youngest member of the Greasers. His closest friend in the Greasers is Johnny, who, as a result of his abusive and rejecting parents, feels more at home in the gang and on the streets than in his own house. It is not unusual for Johnny to leave his house in the evening and sleep in a park to escape the stress in his home life. Johnny becomes the victim of a serious beating by the Socs when he is alone walking in the evening. As a result of this attack, which leaves Johnny scarred and scared, Johnny begins carrying a switchblade.

Following a verbal fight with his brother Darry one evening, Ponyboy runs out of the house to find Johnny. The two decide to stay away from their homes that evening and sleep in the park. During the night, they are jumped by a carload of Socs. As the Socs are holding Ponyboy's head in a fountain "to get the grease off of him," Johnny fears that they are going to drown his friend; Johnny knifes the ringleader of the Socs. The switchblade kills the Soc, and all involved leave the scene in a frenzy. At the advice of another Greaser (Dally) whom they frantically search out that evening, Ponyboy and Johnny jump a train to a neighboring town, where they plan to hide out in an abandoned church until other plans are made.

One evening, the boys are returning to the church when they notice it is on fire. As they run up the hill toward the blaze, they find chaos. A group of small children and adults have been at the church, and several of the children were trapped inside when the fire erupted. The boys run into the church and save the children but sustain serious injuries. Johnny dies as a result of his injuries. The media heralds the boys as heroes.

Tragedy and violence surround the adolescents throughout the book, whether within their homes or on the streets. Two of the main characters die untimely deaths through violent acts. Dally is also killed while attempting to rob a store. The two gangs are involved in street fights, exercising their rights to the street, while family members, parents, and siblings are also involved in verbal and physical fights at home.

Throughout the book, Ponyboy continues to reflect on each incident as it occurs. Through his eyes and his voice, the reader experiences his struggles with his life. It is at the conclusion of the book that Ponyboy resolves to give new meaning to the violence and tragedy in his life. He commits to changing his life.

Not all adolescent readers will identify with all of the aspects of street life as described in this novel. However, it is Ponyboy's struggles, confusion, and decisions that all adolescents, across the typical boundaries of gender, social class, and race, can relate to. Also, the first-person writing style of this novel brings the reader into Ponyboy's world: his thoughts, his needs, his desires, his frustrations. The reader immediately identifies with his loneliness, his confusion, and his desire for a better life.

Lastly, the roles, reactions, and responsibilities of the adults as portrayed by the teacher, the judge, the priest, and the guy who offers Ponyboy a ride provide insight as to how adolescents view the adults in their lives. It is their reactions and support, or lack thereof, that reinforce adolescents' views of themselves as "outsiders" to the adult world.

BASIC NEEDS AND THE CURRENT CONDITION

From the early research of Abraham Maslow (1970), a hierarchy of basic human needs was developed. The needs of food, clothing, shelter safety, security, and a sense of belonging and love set the foundation for this hierarchy. According to this theory, self-actualization of inner talent by maximizing potential through individual achievement and mastery is realized once these foundational needs are met. Current brain research continues to support the theory; responses from those who are fearful and hungry are more protective than from those who are not. The brain's system of automatic response, such as "fight or flight," takes over to protect at times of perceived adversity (Hart, 1983). In other words, it is difficult, if not neurologically impossible, to engage in intellectual pursuits when the most basic needs are unmet. Ponyboy, Darry, Johnny, and the other characters in *The Outsiders* represent youth struggling to fulfill their basic needs. Their most basic of needs—for shelter, belonging, and safety—are not met through the family, school, or church organizations, but through their street gangs. Fearful and hungry, they resort to fights and escapes when challenged with adversity, either at home or on the streets.

Ponyboy, Darry, and Johnny are not alone in representing the needs of children and adolescents in our society. Children and adolescents are thrust into the world of adult decisions. Youth are marrying, producing children, dying, and being left alone at an ever increasing and ever more alarming rate. From research with the Children's Defense Fund, Marian Wright Edelman (1989) concluded, "Millions of children are not safe physically, educationally, economically, or spiritually. The poor black youths who shoot up drugs on street corners and the rich white youths who do the same thing in their mansions share a common disconnectedness from any hope or purpose" (24).

Among adults, however, the argument is frequently made that these issues are greater than the scope of what can be solved by society. Previously, the basic needs of children were primarily addressed through the family, church, and community. However, where and how are these basic needs currently being met for our children? A theme that is glaringly obvious throughout the course of *The Outsiders* is the absence of adult involvement. There are instances in the book where Ponyboy reaches out to the adults in the novel: the man who picks him up following a fight and drops him off at home because the man sees himself as a "good guy"; the juvenile judge who tells Ponyboy to quit biting his nails while the judge is deciding Ponyboy's fate; and the teacher whom Ponyboy calls at home one evening to ask about an assignment. All three of these individuals, representing the systems to support children and youth in our society (the community, the judicial system, and the educational system), fail miserably to meet the needs of a youth calling for help. Each of the adult characters in the book identifies and addresses the immediate needs at a surface level, without going deeper to investigate the real issues and reasons.

Many adults feel overwhelmed by the current needs of our children and youth. But what are the adult responsibilities? How should the adults get in? How do the society and community respond to the changing needs of children and adolescents?

Current Responses

Responses to these issues of changing needs and expectations for children and adolescents depend upon an accurate assessment of the problem within either a reactive or proactive frame of reference. Historically and across disciplines, common responses to these issues all shared the tendency to attribute the problems to the troubled individual. Specifically, this involved the professional reactions of labeling and targeting blame, then combating or disengaging from the individual and the problem. Brendtro, Brokenleg, and Van Bockern (1990) discuss the commonality of responses among professionals to the difficult challenges faced by youth. Across professions, the reactions to challenges have included: identify, label (as disturbed, deprived, dysfunctional, disabled, etc.), and segregate to treat the problem.

The eventual result of these reactive responses to the current issues of the human condition was actually the creation of more negative traits, such as feelings of inferiority, continued lack of safety and belonging, and avoidance, which further exacerbated the issues already faced by the increasingly disrespectful, rejected, and discouraged children and youth (Brendtro, Brokenleg, and Van Bockern, 1990). Kunc (1992) suggests that these responses of eventual rejection and segregation within education (e.g., school suspensions and expulsions, special education, etc.) actually corrupt Maslow's hierarchy of basic needs. These reactive responses demand that children attain achievement, mastery, and positive recognition *before* the children may belong and be included in the family, in the school, or in the community.

Another issue to consider regarding the typical adult responses to current needs is the framing of the perceived needs of youth by adults. The adult reactions to the needs of the adolescents in *The Outsiders* provide examples of solutions to incorrectly defined problems. The teacher does answer her phone, does provide Ponyboy with the information about the assignment, and does address the immediate issue posed by the situation. However, when does the greater question of Ponyboy's poor school attendance get addressed? Who is there for the main characters when the parents tragically die? Who is there to help them when the judge decides their fate? Who helps them when Darry, the older brother, is appointed their custodian? Do any of the adults notice the bruises, scars, and symbols that identify the street gang activity? Are adults content to address the current issues with quick-fix solutions? One of the adult characters in the novel proclaims, "I am one of the good guys" as he drives Ponyboy home from the street fight. Are we, as adults, the "good guys" in the eyes of our children and adolescents?

Proactively Meeting Basic Needs

To counteract reactive, quick-fix responses, it is critical to know the alternatives and proactively plan and implement education responses that address basic needs. Principles of healthy child development, studied across disciplines and centuries (Coopersmith, 1967; Glasser, 1986; Mendler, 1992), focus on four specific human needs. The first of the basic needs is a sense of belonging and connection within a group. Significance is found through the acceptance, attention, and affection of others (Coopersmith, 1967). Competence, the second need, develops as one masters the environment (i.e., successfully masters the academic and behavioral content and expectations at school). Success brings satisfaction and a sense of efficacy whereas chronic failure stifles motivation (Coopersmith, 1967). The ability to control one's own behavior and therefore gain the respect of others develops a sense of control, power, and independence among children. This self-control, the third need, counteracts the negative feelings of helplessness. The last component is the need to contribute through generosity and giving to others. This develops a sense of worthiness. Without feelings of worthiness, life is not fulfilling.

Youth development is an ongoing growth process, in which all youth attempt to meet their basic and social needs to be safe, feel cared for, be valued, be useful, and be spiritually grounded, and in which they strive to build skills and competencies that allow them to function and contribute in their daily lives (Pittman, O'Brien, and Kimball, 1993). This development occurs through interactions within families, peer groups, and communities. Whether youths' needs are met and their skills are used in socially acceptable ways depends, in large part, on the quality and availability of people, places, and possibilities. Young people will seek ways to meet needs and will build and use competencies whether or not these are socially acceptable.

The main characters of *The Outsiders* are constantly struggling to proactively provide for these basic needs. Ponyboy and his brothers, although very different in desires and interests, unite against others. Their brotherly ties and their identification with their street gang provide the sense of connection to a greater source of power. The street gang involvement is a natural extension of the need to belong in a social group when the community, school, and family do not address this need. The fact that Ponyboy's brothers are also part of the gang, combined with the absence of parents (either through death, as in Ponyboy's case, or because parents are emotionally unavailable, as in Johnny's case), further increases the likelihood of gang involvement.

The street rumbles and brawls constantly challenge and exert the need for competence and power over what is in the world of many of the main characters. The streets and those on the streets provide the only venue for competently controlling their world. It is within that venue that two of the characters die asserting their need for power and competence over their world. Although Ponyboy is a part of that world, he also is competent in, and even enjoys, other interests, such as reading and soccer. Competence, at least for Ponyboy, has been in several other arenas in his life.

The need for competence directly relates to the resulting power and self-control one exerts within one's own life. The tragic loss of their parents leaves Ponyboy, Soda, and Darry without a familial sense of identity. Through no one's fault, they are immediately thrust into a world that they now need to control, by independently addressing their own needs. The transition is difficult without adult assistance. The main characters again turn to their peers, their gangs, and their brothers to develop their own sense of control over family and life situations that, at times, leave them feeling very much out of control. Although Ponyboy relies on and loves his brothers, he also exhibits a strong sense of autonomy, from the very outset of the book. He describes himself as a "loner," has interests and needs different from those of his peers, and often seeks solutions different from theirs.

The rescue of the small children during the fire at the abandoned church illustrates the need of the main characters to contribute. Despite the current condition of their own lives and the possible repercussions, Ponyboy, Johnny, and Darry immediately act to save the children. Their sense of purpose and need to contribute transcend any personal needs for comfort, safety, or, in Johnny's case, survival.

Left with a virtual absence of adult guidance, support, or even interaction, the youth of *The Outsiders* interact with their peers to develop and meet their basic needs. The results of their struggles are tragic for several of the main characters. The outcome for Ponyboy's life, however, is the exception among the members of his gang. Although faced with similar issues and conditions, Ponyboy survives and resolves to make some changes in his life. What factors enhance his opportunities for survival? Could what is currently known about the factors of survival be built upon to assist youth development for all children?

YOUTH DEVELOPMENT: DEVELOPING RESILIENCE AMONG CHILDREN AND ADOLESCENTS

Numerous developmental and longitudinal studies have been undertaken to study children and youth at risk from the perspective of survival. In her review of the youth resilience literature, Bonnie Benard (1991) identifies several characteristics among children who from early ages were considered at high risk of developing problems but who grew up to become happy, healthy, productive adults. The first characteristic is social competence. Social competence includes empathy, caring, communication skills, and prosocial behaviors within a social setting. The second characteristic, problem-solving skills, includes the ability to think abstractly, reflectively, and flexibly and to arrive at competent alternative solutions to both cognitive and social problems. A sense of autonomy and identity, coupled with an ability to act independently and exert control over your environment, is the third characteristic. The fourth and last characteristic identified is the sense of purpose and future, including healthy expectations, goal directedness, hopefulness, and a sense of coherence.

In addition, Benard summarizes the protective factors within the family, school, and community that seem to contribute to youth development and resilient children. At all three levels (family, school, and community), the protective factors are the same: a caring and supportive environment; high expectations; and opportunities for meaningful involvement, empowerment, and participation.

FRAMEWORK FOR CHANGE IN EDUCATION

If the role of education is that of the equalizer of the human condition (Little, 1997), the responsibilities and opportunities to enhance youth development are critical and far reaching. Although some of the issues previously discussed appear daunting, Covey (1991) suggests any proactive action plan begins within our circle of influence. Teachers and school personnel possess tremendous opportunities through daily decision making to significantly and permanently impact the current conditions and future development of the children within our classrooms and our schools (Ginott, 1990). In fact, the resolution of some of the major concerns facing our children today depends upon teachers proactively influencing the human condition of the children and youth through their actions within the educational system. Research on effective schools has shown a key characteristic of these schools to be the creation of a proactive, caring school community rather than a series of isolated practices in reaction to current perceived problems (Phi Delta Kappa Commission on Discipline, 1982). Societal institutions serve as powerful environments to transmit societal values, norms, and social mores to the young (Wozner, 1985).

How do adults proactively plan and create caring and responsive communities and services that address the basic needs of healthy youth development? Based upon the four basic developmental needs of all children, the Community Circle of Caring model (Blankstein and De-Four, 1997) provides a specific framework for change. By creating classrooms, schools, and programs around the concepts of connection, competence, self-control, and contribution, adults can create caring classroom and school communities that address the four basic developmental needs of all students within an educational circle of influence.

The first component needed for change is a connection for students. As humans, we want to be connected with something larger, more identifiable, more important than ourselves. The need to be affiliated and connected with a group, whether as members of a street gang or a church choir, begins with the process of welcoming within the group. From the very first day of school, it is critical to include all students as connected members of the total group. Do teachers spend the time to connect students with other students and with adults in the school and classroom? Is there at least one other person who is connected to each of the students? Are the special talents and interests of each member of the class discovered and enhanced within the group? Are identifiable emblems or signs visible to the members of the class or activity group? Is every member of the class or school valued and humanized as a person?

Second, information is power. Within a classroom, competence at academic tasks is critical for each of the students. A grasp of the information and objectives of a particular curriculum provides the power of knowledge. Given the academic needs of students, the expert implementation of numerous, varied pedagogical techniques is a must if teachers are to develop competence within the curriculum for each child in the classroom. The use of researched techniques, such as cooperative learning, mnemonics, advance organizers, active engagement strategies, and classwide peer tutoring, enhances the competence for each student within our classrooms. Further schoolwide strategies, such as after-school tutoring, academic knowledge contests, learning resource centers, and teacher assistance teams, also can enhance the competence of the students. Is each student mastering the curriculum? What strategies and techniques have been implemented to plan for student learning?

Teaching responsibility to students combined with self-control results in the development of responsible, well-disciplined students, not merely obedient students (Kriedler, 1988). Clearly organized and well-communicated expectations and procedures enhance student self-control within the classroom community. Clearly articulating and reinforcing mutually agreed-upon rules and roles for all members of the classroom community provide ownership and a sense of empowerment. Individual growth and continued contribution can occur once the framework for specific expectations has been agreed upon and communicated. Do students clearly understand expectations? Have the procedures been practiced and reinforced? Is the classroom well organized to maximize the teaching and learning process? Have the students had an active role in the development of the procedures of the classroom and the school? Are there natural consequences within the community?

Lastly, engaging, effective classroom communities enhance the contribution of all members (Little, 1997). By knowing each student's strengths, interests, and needs, a teacher can engage students more actively within the learning. By employing various active engagement techniques (e.g., questioning skills, peer partners, classwide peer tutoring, variety of response methods), teachers can increase the frequency of successful student response. Within the school, connecting each student with any one of the numerous school-based activities will increase the opportunity for each student to make a positive contribution to the total school community.

EXPANDING THE CIRCLE

Meeting the needs of some children and youth of today requires more intensive and comprehensive approaches. Teachers and school personnel, in collaboration with families, mental health professionals, peers, and entire communities, can offer numerous educational opportunities to meet basic needs. Several curricula have been developed to work with parents of adolescents who are at risk. (See the recommended readings.) Parents can monitor and regulate their children's behavior through education of both the parent and the child. Social skills training is a critical component. Evaluations of these proactive approaches have suggested that they lead to improvements in family interactions, such as reduced family conflict and improved family organization and cohesion, and to fewer signs of depression, withdrawal, aggressiveness, delinquency, and somatic complaints (Office of Special Education Programs, 1992).

School-based programs often seen as "best-practice" models link mental health treatment programs with classroom instruction for children and adolescents. Pivotal to the operation is intensive personal attention and a supportive network of teachers, counselors, and peers. A three-pronged approach consisting of academics, counseling, and vocational training and placement has resulted in improved outcomes for children and adolescents (Pittman, 1991).

Several studies have described the value of expanding the circle by connecting children and adolescents to their peers. Peer programs that highlight peer influence and emphasize skill development have been found to be the most successful (Tobler, 1986). Peer counseling and student assistance programs offer unique opportunities for youth to cope with difficult issues and develop skills to resist peer pressure (Office of Special Education Programs, 1992; Hawkins, Catalano, and Miller, 1992).

Finally, when considering expanding the circle to proactively reach all children and adolescents, remember that religious organizations, housing and community development organizations, direct-service nonprofit organizations, and businesses exist in all communities. Insufficient attention has been paid to the identification and development of their combined capacity to offer young people the opportunities, structures, and concrete supports and services they need to bring purpose to their present lives as they prepare for their futures.

SUMMARY AND IMPLICATIONS

Today, one in four adolescents in the United States engages in high-risk behaviors that endanger his or her own health and well-being and that of others. We must reach these young people early and provide them with both the means and motivation to avoid risky, destructive activities . . . Unfortunately, too few adults invest the personal time and effort to encourage, guide, and befriend young people who are struggling to develop the skills and confidence necessary for a successful and satisfying adult life. Too few communities encourage and recognize community service by young people. And too few offer programs and activities to promote

healthy adolescent development. . . . As a result, many young people believe they have little to lose by dropping out of school, having a baby as
an unmarried teenager, and committing crimes. (*Beyond Rhetoric*, National
Commission on Children, 1991)

Considering the issues raised in the novel *The Outsiders*, reframing
the needs of all children and youth from a reactive, blame-and-label-the-
victim system to a comprehensive, proactive system of youth development is not a task for the faint of heart. While a popular adage states
that it takes a village to raise a child, in the case of teens such as Ponyboy
and the members of the Greasers, it takes a society and its support systems jumping in and rolling up their sleeves. But the first task is identifying the problem accurately. Does each adult accept the responsibility
of *working* on the problem—the *real* problem? Are adults content to
only respond to the question, if even posed? What could have been
different if adults in Ponyboy's life had rolled up their sleeves at the first
signs of difficulty: his parents' deaths, his increasing truancy, his de-
creasing grades, his changing appearance?

Once a need has been identified, how do we react? Do we blame or
label the student, then dismiss the concerns? Do we ascribe the characteristics of the label to the student? Although Ponyboy was a good student who enjoyed school, the educational system, as seen through his
eyes, was not a welcoming, caring place when he turned to that social
system for support:

> The first week of school after the hearing had been awful. People I knew
> wouldn't talk to me, and people I didn't know would come right up and
> ask about the whole mess. Sometimes even the teachers. And my history
> teacher—she acted as if she was scared of me, even though I'd never
> caused any trouble in her class. You can bet that made me feel real tough.
> (Hinton, 1989, p. 147)

How different Ponyboy's and the Greasers' stories could have been if
adults had not forced them into the role of outsiders!

Successful youth development takes the initiative, effort, and dedication of adults within the community—family members, school personnel,
and community members. This community commitment must be accom-
panied by strong, visible community action to build on the known resilience factors and characteristics for total youth development. The
characters, both youth and adults, in *The Outsiders* provide a glimpse of

the continually worsening condition of our nation's youth. If desired outcomes for today's youth continue to be social and community skills, community commitment, leadership, self-awareness, autonomy, and a sense of future for all youth, there is a need to commit to more and better adult involvement within our communities. The challenges of appropriate youth development for all of our children and youth necessitate action by all adults. The legacy of the American dream can only be preserved for future generations through the continued commitment of the current generation.

RECOMMENDED READINGS

Fiction

London, Jonathan. (1997). *Where's home?* New York: Penguin. 96 pp. (ISBN: 0–140–37513–9). MS.

Adrian is 14 years old and homeless. His father, a Vietnam veteran, has had a hard life. Together, they travel the open road, searching for peace of mind.

McLaughlin, Frank. (1991). *Yukon journey.* New York: Scholastic. 99 pp. (ISBN: 0–590–43538–8). MS.

Sixteen-year-old Andy is bullied at school, but he cannot talk about it with his father, who still blames Andy for the death of their family dog. Andy feels ashamed and afraid of his father's anger. When his dad's plane crashes in the Yukon, he knows that he has to find his father, and Andy embarks on a terrifying journey of self-discovery.

Murphy, Barbara Beasley. (1994). *Fly like an eagle.* New York: Delacorte. 178 pp. (ISBN: 0–385–32035–3). MS, HS.

Traveling from New York to Mexico, Barney and his 17-year-old son, Ace, go looking for Barney's natural father. Not knowing his father was adopted, Ace learns that Barney's life as an orphan mirrors his own quest for self-identity.

O'Neal, Zibby. (1985). *In summer light.* New York: Bantam. 152 pp. (ISBN: 0–553–25940–7). HS.

Kate has always felt overwhelmed by her identity as the daughter of the world-famous painter Marcus Brewer. It is only during her long summer recovering from mononucleosis that Kate begins to confront her feelings about herself, her own art, and her relationship with her celebrated father.

Paulsen, Gary. (1994). *The haymeadow*. New York: Dell. 195 pp. (ISBN: 0–440–40923–3). MS, HS.

Wanting to please an uncaring father is the theme of this novel. John, the son, spends his summer tending six thousand sheep because he hopes to win his father's affection. But, unprepared to deal with a series of natural disasters, John wonders why he ever embarked on this perilous journey.

Pausewang, Gordon. (1994). *Fall-out*. Translated by Patricia Crampton. New York: Viking. 172 pp. (ISBN: 0–670–86104–9). MS.

Fourteen-year-old Janna's life is turned upside down by a nuclear power plant accident. She falls ill with radiation sickness, witnesses an entire countryside contaminated, and challenges the very system that has jeopardized her life.

Peck, Richard. (1996). *Father figure*. New York: Puffin. 208 pp. (ISBN: 0–140–37969–X). MS, HS.

A father shows up unexpectedly at the funeral of his children's mother, leaving his two sons in a quandary. Seventeen-year-old Jim and his younger brother, Bryan, must now live with the father in his Florida home. Sparks fly as father and sons learn to reconcile their anger and pain.

Powell, Randy. (1995). *Dean Duffy*. New York: Farrar, Straus & Giroux. 170 pp. (ISBN: 0–374–31754–2). HS.

When Dean Duffy, star athlete, hits a major slump in his baseball playing right before high school graduation, he is forced to examine what he really wants to do with sports and his future.

Pringle, Terry. (1988). *The preacher's boy*. Carrabo, NC: Algonquin. 280 pp. (ISBN: 0–192–6977–6). MS, HS.

Michael is the son of a preacher and is usually at odds with his father's puritanical teachings. Going away to college does not help when his father learns that Michael has moved in with his girlfriend Amy.

Rodowsky, Colby. (1985). *Julie's daughter*. New York: Farrar, Straus & Giroux. 231 pp. (ISBN: 0–374–33963–5). HS.

Julie's daughter, nicknamed Slug, has lived with her grandmother for seventeen years. Suddenly, Slug's grandmother dies, and Slug accepts an offer to live with her real mother, Julie. The move, though, proves traumatic as mother and daughter—never friends—struggle to reconcile their ever present anger and distrust.

Nonfiction

Bauman, Lawrence, and Robert Riche. (1987). *The nine most troublesome teenage problems*. New York: Ballantine. 289 pp. (ISBN: 0–345–34290–9). HS.

This is a highly readable presentation of the nine most common problems that parents encounter with teenagers: sex, loneliness, lying, boredom, bad school performance, no communication, anger, hanging out with a bad crowd, and irresponsibility.

Eyre, Richard, and Linda Eyre. (1994). *Three steps to a strong family*. New York: Simon & Schuster. 235 pp. (ISBN: 0–671–88728–9). HS.

This helpful guide for raising responsible young people and making families strong and healthy features practical advice and hands-on exercises.

Goleman, Daniel. (1997). *Emotional intelligence: Why it can matter more than IQ*. New York: Bantam. 352 pp. (ISBN: 0–553–37506–7). HS.

Goleman demonstrates that many factors can influence success—beside IQ. These factors include self-awareness, self-discipline, and empathy, and add up to a different way of being smart.

REFERENCES

Annie E. Casey Foundation. (1996). *Kids count data book: State profiles of child well-being*. Baltimore, MD: Annie E. Casey Foundation.

Benard, B. (1991). *Fostering resiliency in kids: Protective factors in the family, school, and community*. San Francisco: Western Regional Center for Drug-Free Schools and Communities.

Blankstein, A., and R. DeFour. (1997). *Reaching today's students: Building the community circle of caring*. Bloomington, IN: National Educational Service.

Brendtro, L., M. Brokenleg, and S. Van Bockern. (1990). *Reclaiming youth at risk: Our hope for the future*. Bloomington, IN: National Educational Service.

Coopersmith, S. (1967). *The antecedents of self-esteem*. New York: Perennial.

Covey, S. (1991). *Principle-centered leadership*. New York: Simon & Schuster.

Edelman, M. (1989). Children at risk. *Proceedings of the Academy of Political Science* 27 (2): 20–30.

Ginott, H. (1990). *Teacher and child*. New York: Simon & Schuster.

Glasser, W. (1986). *Control theory in the classroom*. New York: Harper & Row.

Hart, L. (1983). *Human brain and human learning*. New York: Longman.

Hawkins, J. D., R. Catalano, and J. Miller. (1992). Risk and protective factors for alcohol and other drug problems in adolescence and early adulthood: Implications for substance abuse prevention. *Psychological Bulletin* 112 (1): 64–105.

Hinton, S. E. (1989). *The outsiders*. New York: Dell.

Kozol, J. (1995). *Savage inequalities*. New York: Crown.

Kriedler, C. (1988). *Resolving conflicts in schools*. Boston: Allyn & Bacon.

Kunc, N. (1992). *The corruption of Maslow's hierarchy*. New York: Axis Consultation and Training.

Little, M. (1997). *Teaching our students: Building a community circle of caring*. Bloomington, IN: National Educational Service.

Maslow, A. (1970). *Motivation and personality*. New York: Harper & Row.

Mendler, A. (1992). *What do I do when . . . ?: How to achieve discipline with dignity in the classroom*. Bloomington, IN: National Educational Service.

National Commission on Children. (1991). *Beyond rhetoric*. Washington, DC: National Commission on children.

Office of Special Education Programs. (1992). *Signs of effectiveness: The high-risk youth demonstration grants*. Rockville, MD: Office of Special Education Programs.

Phi Delta Kappa Commission on Discipline. (1982). *Handbook for developing schools with good discipline*. Bloomington, IN: Phi Delta Kappa Commission on Discipline.

Pittman, K. (1991). *A new vision: Promoting youth development*. Oak Brook, IL: Center for Youth Development and Policy Research.

Pittman, K., R. O'Brien, and M. Kimball. (1993). *Youth development and resiliency research: Making connections to substance abuse prevention*. San Francisco: Western Regional Center for Drug-Free Schools and Communities.

Tobler, N. (1986). Meta analysis of 143 adolescent drug prevention programs: Quantitative outcome results of program participants compared to a control or comparison group. *Journal of Drug Issues* 16 (4): 537–567.

Wozner, Y. (1985). Institution as community. *Child and Youth Services* 7: 71–90.

CHAPTER 8

Identity Confusion: Zibby O'Neal's *The Language of Goldfish*

Marcia F. Nash and David B. Daniel

INTRODUCTION

The time between ages 9 and 14 is a period when humans begin the journey from childhood through adolescence to adulthood. The physical changes that begin during this time are predictable and universal. Although we pass through the changes—in body shape, skin, hair, and hormones—at different rates and to varying degrees, puberty is an observable, biological process. Adolescence is much more complicated. It encompasses physical, social, and cognitive development. All of this development takes place in a cultural context that offers complex, and sometimes contradictory, expectations, values, and models of psychological health. Identity conflict/confusion is relatively common during early adolescence. For some, it is a time to begin the search for the "right mask." But others will take an active part in their own development and grow beyond the need for a mask.

Carrie Stokes, the protagonist in Zibby O'Neal's novel *The Language of Goldfish* is teetering on the edge of her childhood. At 13, she is beyond the boundaries of childhood as they are defined in her insulated, upper-middle-class community and by her family. Carrie and her family moved to Northpoint, an exclusive suburb of Chicago, when Carrie's father finished medical school and began his private practice. Carrie's mother has taken on the role of suburban housewife, running the house with the help of a maid and trying to provide her children with the skills and the tools they need to survive in their new environment. Carrie's 15-year-old sister, Moira, has moved smoothly from Chicago to Northpoint and from childhood to adolescence. Moira seems perfectly at home in the world of school dances and double dates. Duncan, Carrie's younger brother, still lives in a world of soccer games and Saturday matinees. As Carrie moves through her eighth-grade year, she feels herself being plucked out of childhood and dropped into adolescence. All the expectations and role changes brought on by adolescence terrify Carrie. As Carrie clings to her childhood, she suffers a crisis that makes her question who she is and who she must become.

SYNOPSIS

It is in September of her eighth-grade year at Sylvester Country Day School that Carrie Stokes first starts experiencing symptoms of her illness. As Carrie gets ready for school one morning, her mother tries to give her a check to pay for attendance at the school dances. When Carrie refuses, her mother reminds her that Moira had loved the dances. Carrie in turn reminds her mother that she is not Moira. That's when it happens for the first time.

> It was curiously hard to explain what had happened. In a way, it didn't seem like much of anything. A dizzy spell. But at the same time Carrie had known from the beginning, without really knowing, that it was something worse than being dizzy. (11)

It becomes clear to Carrie that Moira agrees with their parents. It is time for Carrie to leave her childhood behind. One morning on the way to school, Moira warns Carrie that she "can't go on being a little kid forever" (13). Carrie feels dizzy again. Moira's opinion is particularly important to Carrie. They had been close as children and had even shared a special fantasy. When the girls first moved to the house in Northpoint, they discovered a pond. When the girls threw crackers into the pond and whistled, goldfish appeared. They had discovered the language of goldfish. But even as Moira engaged in the fantasy play, she was already moving out of her childhood, and away from the place that Carrie very much wanted to stay.

Although Carrie does well in school, she doesn't like it. She doesn't seem to fit in. Mrs. Ramsay is really the only friend that Carrie has. Her private art lessons on Saturday morning with Mrs. Ramsay keep Carrie going during the week.

As the school year progresses, Carrie begins to think more about the school dances, which are held at the Northpoint Club. The last day to sign up approaches, and Carrie has still not given her mother's check to the school secretary. Carrie begins to panic. When Carrie tries to discuss her fear of the dances with Moira, Moira responds by saying that it is no big deal, that *everybody* goes to the eighth-grade dances. She informs Carrie that to not go to the dances is weird.

When Carrie finally makes up her mind to try to go to the dance, and gives her money to the school secretary, she has another episode of her illness. This time it is more than dizziness. Her head grows light. Her vision and hearing become distorted into a form of chaos. Then, out of the chaos, "all at once, a bit of land—a sunny, quiet rock—floated up, bobbed, and disappeared" (39).

As Carrie's episodes increase in severity, she begins to wonder if she is going crazy. When she tries to explain to her father what she is going through, he tells her that she has grown a great deal and is probably anemic. Her mother tells her that all she needs is more rest and a proper breakfast. Carrie can't make anyone understand what she is experiencing.

After a particularly terrifying episode, in which she finds herself wandering on the edge of town with hours of her life a complete blank, Carrie gives in to the chaos and the lure of the island. She goes into the bathroom and takes an overdose of pills.

After her suicide attempt, Carrie is hospitalized for a month. When she returns home, her family welcomes her, but they want to go on with their lives and want Carrie to get on with hers. Her mother refers to Carrie's suicide attempt as "an unfortunate incident" (82).

Carrie continues to see Dr. Ross, a therapist who began working with her in the hospital. And she very slowly returns to her art and her work with Mrs. Ramsay. Her art begins to change. Carrie becomes concerned that she has killed off the part of herself that could draw, but Mrs. Ramsay assures her that her current drawings are "marking-time pictures" (115). Carrie's art is as transitional as her life.

Carrie begins to take tentative steps into adolescence. She asks Moira to buy her a bra. She begins a friendship with Daniel, her new neighbor and a fellow advanced math student. And she begins to draw, and then paint, the island she had seen during her episodes. Carrie also makes another attempt to explain to Moira her fears, her confusion, and her reluctance to change.

"Moira, don't you still kind of believe in the fish language—even though you're older now?"
"No. I tell you that every time you ask."

"Did you stop a very long time ago?"

"Ages ago."

Carrie felt questions struggling inside her. She didn't know how to ask them. She leaned forward. Her voice became urgent, too high.

"Do I have to stop Moira?" she cried. "Do I *have* too?"

Moira looked at her. "You *know* it was a game," Moira said.

"But I want to believe it! I don't want to lose everything!"

"Lose what?" Moira said. "What do you mean by everything?"

Carrie drew in her breath and shook her head, "I can't explain." (141)

Throughout her hospitalization and months of after-school therapy, Carrie and her family keep her illness and suicide attempt a secret. But after an encounter with an unpleasant girl in one of her classes, Carrie realizes that others must wonder where she goes every day after school, why she doesn't go to the dances, and why she doesn't have any friends. She decides that she will go to the last dance of the year so that the other kids won't think of her as a "creep" anymore.

Carrie survives the dance and the eighth grade. She spends the following summer working, drawing, and thinking about what has happened to her. By August, when Dr. Ross goes away on vacation, she feels strong. When she starts therapy again in the fall, she feels that she has begun to figure out what has happened to her. She comes to the realization that she's never liked change and that growing up was a huge change she had pretended would never happen. Finally, she can no longer pretend.

When Carrie returns home from her session with Dr. Ross, a young neighbor, Sara Meyers, has come to visit. Carrie takes Sara to the pond and teaches her about the language of goldfish. Sara thinks it is magic. As Carrie watches Sara play at the edge of the pond, she sees for the first time that the island in the middle of the pond is the same island that she saw when she hallucinated during her illness, and it is the same island that she has been drawing. Carrie wonders why it has taken her so long to recognize it. She realizes that it is a very small island and that she could reach it easily with the handle of a broom.

CARRIE'S JOURNEY FROM CHILDHOOD TO ADOLESCENCE

Carrie's journey from childhood to adolescence is certainly a perilous one. Although most children don't experience early adolescence in as

extreme a way as Carrie does, many do experience similar fears, frustrations, and questions about who they are and who they are becoming.
In this section of the chapter, we use Carrie's experiences to explore the
physical, cognitive, and social development of early adolescence.

Physical Development

At the beginning of the book, Carrie has a childlike disinterest in her
appearance and her body. She passively submits to critiques of her hair
and clothing by her mother and Moira.

As Carrie's awareness of her physical self increases, so does her distress. After her suicide attempt, Carrie realizes that her body is changing
and that she cannot stop the changes from happening. During a bath,
Carrie becomes acutely aware of her lack of control over her own body.

The adolescent growth spurt is a period of rapid growth resulting in
increased height, weight, and body shape. While individual differences
do occur among females, the growth spurt occurs approximately two
years prior to first menstruation, or menarche. The average white American middle- to upper-middle-class female begins her adolescent growth
spurt about age 11 (Malina, 1991) and achieves menarche between 12
and 13 years of age (Eveleth and Tanner, 1978). Breast budding and
development usually occur prior to this age as well.

According to these averages, Carrie is slightly behind the average female at her school with respect to physical development. At 13 years of
age, she is just beginning to develop breasts and has yet to have her first
menstrual period. The psychological effects of later development are
minimal for females and not especially useful to consider in Carrie's
case since she is not distressed at being later than others. Rather, Carrie's
obsession is with the *meaning* of these changes and how they will affect
her concept of who she is.

Cognitive Development

Cognitively, Carrie has achieved a level of development consonant
with her age. Piaget's theory predicts that adolescents will become capable of abstract reasoning in the stage of formal operations. The adolescent begins to shift from relying on actual outcomes (based on past
experiences) of events to all of the possible outcomes. Carrie demonstrates her capacity for abstract reasoning, particularly in art and math.

While visiting the art exhibit, Carrie demonstrates her ability to go beyond the concrete.

Research subsequent to Piaget's has questioned whether the attainment of formal operations is universal among adolescents (Flavell, 1985). If this is the case, Carrie's attainment of formal operational thinking would separate her from the majority of her peers, contributing to her feeling of isolation and difference. Carrie's placement in an advanced math class sets her apart from the average students and, in a way, puts her in conflict with the expectations of her community and her family. When Carrie explains to her father that she is late arriving at his office for a ride home because she has been helping a girl at her school with math, her father is not surprised to hear that the girl is not good at math.

Elkind (1966) points out some of the peculiarities of developing abstract thought at an age when personality development is blossoming. By focusing formal operational reasoning on one's own thoughts and behaviors, especially without the benefit of peers for reality testing, the child can become egocentric. One way egocentrism can be manifested is in a feeling that an imaginary audience is always watching the adolescent (Elkind, 1966). The adolescent begins to behave as though every action and thought is the object of others' attention. This is one explanation for the extreme self-consciousness of many adolescents.

While not very concerned about her physical appearance, Carrie is manifesting this form of adolescent egocentrism when she assumes that what she is feeling inside is what everyone else feels about her as well. By projecting her insecurities onto multiple people around her, she initiates a vicious cycle in which she feels like a "loser" and assumes everyone else must feel the same about her, thus compounding and reinforcing her original feelings. Again, without the availability of an actual audience (friend, peer group, sibling, parent, etc.), such a cycle can quickly become self-fulfilling.

Carrie's advanced stage of cognitive development allows her to formulate multiple, and often scary, theories of potential outcomes. She is drowning in a sea of possibilities by thinking hypothetically. Combined with her egocentrism and isolation, this sets the stage for her panic attacks. A child who is not capable of abstract thought would be constrained by the models around her and not able to fully consider the possible alternative outcomes.

Social Development

In general, peer groups dominate early adolescent life. Gender differences in peer groups reflect differences in number and intensity. Females in this age group tend to have smaller peer groups with more intensive emotional intimacy and self-disclosure than do males (Bukatko and Daehler, 1998).

Peer acceptance and status are not of much importance to Carrie. Being neither actively liked nor disliked by her peers, she clearly fits into the category of the peer-neglected child (Asher and Dodge, 1986). A peer-neglected child is one who makes few or no overtures to other children and responds weakly, if at all, to overtures from other children. Consequently, and by mutual agreement, the peer groups do not incorporate this child into their activities. It is as though they do not exist to each other. When Carrie finally attends the dreaded school dance, she has just such an experience: "Carrie looked at . . . the kids straggling in through the doors, joining into groups and laughing. She recognized them all. Nobody noticed. She stood by herself against the wall and watched as if she were watching a play" (156). Research on neglected children does not indicate long-term negative outcomes as it does for children who approach, but are actively rejected by, their peers. This is probably because the child does not desire admittance into a peer group. In Carrie's case, the mutual isolation seems to set the stage for her self-absorption and escalation of symptoms.

Carrie is atypical with respect to social development. Whereas most 13-year-old girls have at least a few close friendships with peers, Carrie seems to have none. At a time when she is going through the traditional struggle of defining who she is and who she may become, Carrie has no one her own age to talk to about what she is feeling and, therefore, has no reality base to gauge if her feelings and reactions are normal. Carrie's older sister, Moira, seems to have moved from childhood to adolescence seamlessly, so it is not surprising that Carrie's few attempts at discussing her feelings with Moira are not very reassuring.

Without the external feedback of reality from her peers, the adolescent can become obsessed, or even lost, in feelings that have been exaggerated by such isolated introspection and self-preoccupation. The absence of social contact is a feature indicative of Carrie's psychological isolation. It sets the stage for exaggerating the importance of what she is going through and exacerbating her feelings of separateness and being "weird."

IDENTITY FORMATION AND IDENTITY CONFUSION

The crisis of adolescence that Erikson (1968) describes is between identity formation and identity confusion. The task for this stage of development is to solidify important elements of identity from childhood and form a clear sense of personal identity. This crisis is a process that can lead from a premature selection of a preexisting role to, as in Carrie's case, identity confusion. Adolescents in a state of identity confusion may exhibit a prolonged period without any commitment to a particular role (Douvan and Adelson, 1971). Their relationships are often superficial and, though they report less closeness and more dissatisfaction with their parents, they have a difficult time determining a sense of personal identity separate from their parents (Conger and Galambos, 1997).

In particular, Carrie's source of confusion revolves around her emerging identity as a woman. While gender identity, the awareness of one's biological gender, is achieved early in life (Huston, 1983), people who are uncomfortable with their sexual nature or reproductive capabilities have a very difficult time during the rapid physical changes of adolescence. In conjunction with Carrie's isolation from peers, this confusion magnifies into genuine panic when she is confronted with stimuli of a sexual or sensual nature.

Carrie has no external outlet for her feelings and no safe place to go. It makes sense that her angst manifests itself in acute anxiety or panic attacks.

CONCLUSION

Carrie is noticing her body changing. She is using this concrete manifestation as a final sign that she cannot remain a child and must embark on a journey into uncharted territory. For many young women, connection with mother or peers allows them to feel that this new territory is not totally unknown. However, Carrie is not close to her mother and has no friends with whom she can discuss this or test reality. Further, the females around her who have taken this journey have, in her eyes, become shallow and self-involved. She does not want this outcome for herself. Therefore, she is taking this journey alone.

Her primary concerns are continuity and predictability. Will she still be Carrie or will she become lost in a rush of hormones and social expectations? This is evident when she notices that tracks in the snow can completely disappear. "The fact that something could vanish entirely was terrifying" (55). Will these changes mean that she will lose herself as the tracks in the snow suggest? The tracks are analogous to her child self.

Carrie's quest to integrate who she thinks she is with who she may become is extremely unsettling to her. With the benefits of an adult role model, friendships, and a peer group, and without the complications of abstract reasoning, Moira's transition was much smoother and more typical. Carrie does not avail herself of these resources. However, as Carrie's ability to think abstractly interacts with the evolution of her concept of self, she begins to take an active role in her own development.

The therapist provides Carrie with the one thing that she thinks she has lost but that she desperately needs: time. Time to become who she will be. Time to allow things to happen. With time Carrie's body will change, and with time Carrie will naturally tire of childish things like space movies, ice forts, and the language of goldfish. With no one pushing her, she will get there herself, in her own time.

Moira's admonition is appropriate: "Let her do it her own way, Mother" (156).

RECOMMENDED READINGS

Fiction

Bennett, James. (1990). *I can hear the morning dove*. New York: Scholastic. 196 pp. (ISBN: 0–590–16309–4). HS.

Since Grace's father died, she has been spiraling out of control. Some days she goes "flat out," only able to sit and cry like a baby. Some nights the nightmares return. How will Grace ever determine who she is or who she wants to be, when reality seems so transitory, so fleeting?

Cormier, Robert. (1991). *I am the cheese*. New York: Bantam Doubleday Dell. 224 pp. (ISBN: 0–685–01413–4). HS.

Adam Farmer is on a journey to find his father. But it is a journey that will never end for Adam because it is a journey into the past. If Adam discovers who he really is and what is buried in his subconscious, he may not survive.

Klass, Sheila. (1995). *Next stop: Nowhere*. New York: Scholastic. 181 pp. (ISBN: 0–590–46686–0). HS.

Fourteen-year-old Beth has lived in New York City with her wealthy mother since her parents divorced. When Beth's mother gets remarried, she sends Beth to Vermont to live with her artist father. Beth must deal with a totally new lifestyle and figure out which of each of her parents' values she will embrace as she moves toward adulthood.

Lutzeier, Elizabeth. (1991). *The wall*. New York: Holiday House. 153 pp. (ISBN: 0–8234–0987–2). HS.

Hannah lives in the shadow of the Berlin Wall. Everything in her world is shrouded in secrecy. When Hannah's mother is shot trying to cross the border, Hannah realizes that she does not even fully know her own parents, or herself.

Martin, Nora. (1997). *The eagle's shadow*. New York: Scholastic. 176 pp. (ISBN: 0–590–36087–6). MS, HS.

Clearie's father has been emotionally distant since his wife, Clearie's mother, left them. When her father must go away for his job, he sends Clearie to live temporarily with her mother's family in a remote Alaskan village. As Clearie learns about her Tlingit heritage, she also learns about her mother and begins to define herself as a person who is really a product of two cultures.

Mazer, Norma. (1990). *C, my name is Cal*. New York: Scholastic. 131 pp. (ISBN: 0–590–41832–7). MS, HS.

Cal feels that there is a piece missing from his life, from his identity. Since Cal's father left years ago, Cal has wondered where his father is and who his father really is. When his father does show up, Cal has to decide how this puzzle piece fits into his vision of who he is and what his life is all about.

Morris, Winifred. (1996). *Liar*. New York: Walker. 161 pp. (ISBN: 0–8027–461–5). MS, HS.

Alex is 14. He is both troubled and in trouble. His life with his mother has taught him to lie, cheat, and steal to survive. When the court system gives Alex one more chance by placing him with his grandparents in a ranching community, Alex discovers that he both wants and needs to change to straighten out his life.

Silvey, Anita. (1997). *Help wanted: Short stories about young people working*. Boston: Little, Brown. 174 pp. (ISBN: 0–316–79148–2). MS, HS.

This collection of a dozen short stories explores the world of teenagers at work. It is a diverse collection by such authors as Gary Soto, Norma Fox Mazer, Ray Bradbury, and Michael Dorris.

Wilson, Budge. (1992). *The leaving and other stories*. New York: Philomel. 207 pp. (ISBN: 0–399–21878–5). MS, HS.

This beautifully crafted collection of short stories features nine young women moving from adolescence to adulthood. Each chronicles her self-discovery as she searches for her place in a complicated world.

Wolff, Virginia Euwer. (1988). *Probably still Nick Swansen*. New York: Scholastic. 175 pp. (ISBN: 0–590–43146–3). MS, HS.

Nick Swansen is a "special ed" kid from room 19. He is very good at some things, like science, but many things are hard for Nick. Shana is a former classmate who has been mainstreamed back into regular classes. At Shana's "going up" party to celebrate her move out of room 19, Nick realizes that he has special feelings for Shana and that she might have special feelings for him. After their date for the prom ends in disaster, the conflict between Nick's limitations and longing to be like everyone else leaves him wondering exactly who he is.

Nonfiction

Atkin, S. Beth. (1996). *Voices from the streets: Young former gang members tell their stories*. Boston: Little, Brown. 131 pp. (ISBN: 0–316–05634–0). MS, HS.

Using interviews, photographs, poems, scrapbooks, and journals, Atkins provides young former gang members with a chance to tell their stories in their own voices. They describe the search for respect, belonging, and safety that got them into gangs, and the search for a new identity and a new life that got them out.

Hoose, Phillip. (1993). *It's our world, too!: Stories of young people who are making a difference*. Boston: Little, Brown. 166 pp. (ISBN: 0–316–37241–2). MS, HS.

Here are the stories of fourteen young activists who are making a difference by actively taking a stand for something they believe in. The book also includes a handbook section that will be helpful to any reader who is ready to make a change in his or her life and world.

Johnson, Andrea. (1997). *Girls speak out: Finding your true self*. New York: Scholastic. 210 pp. (ISBN: 0–316–5634–0). MS, HS.

It is widely believed that girls begin to lose their self-esteem when they reach adolescence. This book is a personal guide to self-esteem for girls age 9 to 14. It is based on workshops Johnson developed for girls and women around the country.

Krementz, Jill. (1989). *How it feels to fight for your life*. Boston: Little, Brown. 132 pp. (ISBN: 0–316–50364–9). ES, MS, HS.

These are the stories of fourteen children, ranging in age from 7 to 16, who face serious illness, disabilities, and traumas. They must deal with surgeries, implants, chemotherapy, medication, and extended hospital stays while also dealing with sibling rivalry, friends, and parents as other children do. What they have in common is a need to find and keep an identity that goes beyond their particular challenge.

Piper, Mary. (1994). *Reviving Ophelia: Saving the selves of adolescent girls*. New York: Random House. 304 pp. (ISBN: 0–345–39282–5). MS, HS, A.

Piper explores the "danger zone" that adolescence, particularly early adolescence, has become for girls in our culture. In clear, jargon-free language, she calls on her years as a therapist, and the stories of girls themselves, to provide a guide for parents, teachers, and therapists as they work with girls and young women moving into adulthood with their "selves" intact.

REFERENCES

Asher, S. R., and K. A. Dodge. (1986). The identification of socially rejected children. *Developmental Psychology* 22: 444–449.

Black, B. (1995). Separation anxiety disorder and panic disorder. In J. S. March (Ed.), *Anxiety disorders in children and adolescents*, New York: Guilford, 212–234.

Bukatko, D., and M. W. Daehler. (1998). *Child development: A thematic approach*, 3rd ed. Boston: Houghton Mifflin.

Conger, J. J., and N. L. Galambos. (1997). *Adolescence and youth: Psychological development in a changing world*, 5th ed. New York: Longman.

Douvan, E., and J. Adelson. (1971). *The adolescent experience*. New York: Wiley.

Elkind, D. (1966). Conceptual orientation shifts in children and adolescents. *Understanding adolescence*. Boston: Allyn & Bacon, 128–158.

Erikson, E. H. (1968). *Identity: Youth and crisis*. New York: Norton.

Eveleth, P., and J. Tanner. (1978). *Worldwide variation in human growth*. Cambridge, MA: Cambridge University Press.

Flavell, J. H. (1985). *Cognitive development*, 2nd ed. Englewood Cliffs, NJ: Prentice-Hall.

Huston, A. C. (1983). Sex typing. In E. M. Hetherington (Ed.) and P. H. Mussen (Series Ed.), *Handbook of child psychology, vol. 4: Socialization, personality, and social development*, 4th ed. New York: Wiley, 387–467.

Malina, R. M. (1991). Growth spurt, adolescence. In R. M. Lerner, A. C. Petersen, and J. Brooks-Gunn (Eds.), *Encyclopedia of adolescence*, vol. 1, New York: Garland.

O'Neal, Zibby. (1980). *The Language of Goldfish*. New York: Viking.

CHAPTER 9

Identity through the Realization of Prejudice: Carolyn Meyer's *Drummers of Jericho*

Tanna M. Gartside and Kristen Sternberg

INTRODUCTION AND SYNOPSIS

Growing up in the nineties is challenging for all adolescent girls, but for Jewish girls the challenge may be greater. As Kaplan (1994) says, "Just as they are coming to terms with who they are emotionally, they often must come to terms with who they are spiritually. Many Jewish teenagers are forced at a young age to define who they are in reference to everyone else" (287). Pazit Trujillo, protagonist in *Drummers of Jericho*, exemplifies this identity dilemma. Pazit, age 14, expected to have a better life in the southern United States town of Jericho with her father, her stepmother, Ellen, and her stepbrothers, Brian and Matt, ages 4 and 6. Pazit and her natural mother had been in conflict for so long that she was not feeling the least bit guilty about leaving Denver and her mother's home. She had come to the new town expecting to have many friends, get to know her father and his new family, do well academically, play in the band, and enjoy a normal high school lifestyle. Instead, her Jewish faith quickly brought her into conflict with the town's Protestant fundamentalism. Pazit's optimism ends abruptly as she becomes the target of religious prejudice that forces her to examine her beliefs and values. In the transition, Pazit learns to come to terms with her own identity and realizes that her faith is more important to her than her petty conflicts with her mother. She returns to her mother's house having learned much about herself.

Pazit thought that a year away from her mother Ruth would have taught the two to relate more effectively. She and Ruth seemed to fight about everything. Therefore, Pazit had been relieved when it came time to depart for her adventure in Israel. For a whole year she had lived, worked, and attended school at a kibbutz with other young Jewish people. However, when the year was over and Pazit returned to her mother's home in Denver, the old conflicts with her mother resumed. Before long, Pazit had petitioned her mother to let her move in with her father, her new stepmother, and her two young stepbrothers in a new town and state. At the end of her fourteenth summer, Pazit moved into her father's home in Jericho.

Just before the school year begins, Pazit becomes acquainted with Billy, an age peer and her first friend in town. Their friendship seems promising, and Pazit is confident that she will have a smooth transition into the new school and the community. What Pazit hasn't anticipated is that Jericho is a closely knit community whose residents are deeply, actively committed to their fundamentalist Protestant faith. Her naïveté carries her into the first day of school, but on that day only hours pass before Pazit is made to realize that her style of dress, her hair style and color, and her complexion are markedly different from those of her classmates. To Pazit, these problems do not seem insurmountable, but in band class she learns that the bandleader has planned a routine for the football game's halftime program in which band members will play Christian hymns and form a cross as they march. Pazit explains to the bandleader that she finds the routine objectionable because it compromises her religious beliefs, but he perceives Pazit's objections as a threat to what he considers a prize-winning routine and succeeds in uniting the other band members against Pazit. "Now Pazit is hurt, scared, angry, and worst of all alone" (93).

Pazit directs her hurt and anger toward her mother, her father, and her father's new family, blaming them all for the sequence of events (the divorce, the remarriage, the move) that led to her presence in this new town. However, she is not willing to talk to her parents directly about this or about problems at school, and she pretends to them that everything is going well.

At school her peers ignore her. Even Billy, whom she had trusted to be her friend, lacks the courage to stand up to his peers, and he pretends not to know her. At home, Pazit's stepmother forgets to respect Pazit's need for kosher menus at mealtimes and calls her by the childish nickname "Zeetie."

When Pazit finally confides in her father about the bandleader's planned program, he offers to talk to the bandleader and promises that he will not bring attention to her while investigating the problem. Rather than feeling relieved, Pazit fears that her father's interventions, no matter how well intended, will cause her more harassment.

Pazit's attempt to handle the conflict between her beliefs and the bandleader's planned routine results in a mutually satisfactory understanding. Pazit will play along with the band, standing on the sidelines of the field while her classmates do the cross formation. Her self-esteem briefly swells, and she is able to approach her stepmother about the kosher meals and the childish nickname.

Billy begins to appear a traitor in Pazit's eyes. The pressure from the bandleader, for whom Billy has a lot of respect, and from his peers is too much for him, and he continues to ignore Pazit publicly. However, his interest in her has privately planted in him a seed, an inkling that there may be a world beyond that of Jericho. He begins to find fault with his girlfriend Tanya's narrow interests. He also speaks about his feelings to his church's youth group leader, but rather than finding encouragement there, Billy is advised to try to convert Pazit to Protestantism.

Then Pazit's father breaks his promise to keep things quiet. His need to resolve what he sees as a civil rights issue leads him to contact the American Civil Liberties Union (ACLU), and Pazit realizes that the situation is out of her hands.

The problems at school escalate. Pazit's classmates become bolder with their taunts as anger replaces curiosity. She becomes the target of name calling and physical threats. Verbal slurs directed at Pazit refer openly to her religious beliefs. Pazit begins to feel sick from stress and makes overtures to one or two of her teachers, but she finds no support. Eventually, her stress symptoms lead her—especially during the time band class meets—to the school nurse, Mrs. Wells.

In the meantime, the ACLU's actions have attracted the notice of the school's parent body, They organize a public forum to speak in favor of the bandleader's right to lead a religious program during the football game's halftime show. Overwhelmingly, the community supports the bandleader at this forum. Billy's mother has forced him to attend the forum and expects him to speak up for the bandleader, as she has. When pressured to speak, however, Billy surprises everyone at the meeting, including himself, as he publicly supports Pazit's right to her beliefs. The entire town begins to turn against Billy, who now feels he has some understanding of Pazit's feelings of alienation.

The bandleader bows to pressure from the ACLU and the media and creates a new routine for the marching band. Pazit then decides to join the band for their entire routine. But she has lost valuable practice time, and her mistakes give her classmates fuel for their taunts against her. The situation culminates with a beautifully wrapped package delivered to her home, containing a dead rat. She accepts defeat and discontinues marching, playing instead from the stands during the opening game. As Rosh Hashanah draws nearer, Pazit makes the decision to return to Denver and celebrate the High Holy Days with her mother. Just before Pazit's departure, Billy makes a public tribute to her at the all-important football game by blatantly leaving the marching band's formation. He marches to where Pazit is sitting and beats a drum solo, shouting, "Hey, Pazit! . . . Listen to my drum solo! I'm dedicating it to you!" (298).

Pazit's return to Denver turns out to last longer than just through the holiday. In a letter to Billy she writes of her somewhat stabilized relationship with her mother, and she discusses her experiences in Jericho from a perspective improved by distance. Billy, in turn, replies with the news that he has been sent to a town not far from Jericho to live with relatives and finish high school there. The two youths vow to continue writing and express their desire to meet again when they are older.

THE PSYCHOLOGICAL PERSPECTIVE

For most adolescents, identity development is a gradual process. During the middle school years the adolescent may overidentify with peers and move away from parents. Early in high school the adolescent starts the search for his or her individual identity and may try on various roles related to political stands, religious issues, career commitments, and romantic involvements. In later adolescence, the youth may become more introspective and search for answers to such questions as, Who am I? What do I believe? Where am I going?

Parental involvement is essential if the adolescent is to reach his or her potential during this developmental quest for identity. But sometimes a parent overidentifies with the adolescent and may feel alienated when the child does not wish to follow the course of action originally planned. At other times a parent may want to control the child and rushes in to rescue when failure seems imminent.

Helping an adolescent develop an identity can take many forms. Being available when needed, but staying in the background, is one form. Pointing out strengths instead of emphasizing weaknesses is a good place to start. Encouraging the child to be involved in extracurricular activities will help develop life skills as well as allow the child to explore career possibilities. When an adolescent makes a statement such as, "I don't know what I want to do in the future," this is generally a cry for help. For an adolescent, having too many interests is normal and healthy. When the child has no hobbies, activities, or interest in the future, the parent need to explore the possibility that the child is suffering from depression.

According to Steinberg and Levine (1990), a parent should be concerned if an identity crisis is:

- *Acute*: The teenager is not just worried about who he or she is, but seriously distressed.
- *Pervasive*: The teenager's distress extends to three or more of the following areas: long-term goals, career choices, friendship patterns, sexuality, religious identity, moral values, group loyalties.
- *Paralyzing*: The teenager is so obsessed with identity questions that he or she performs poorly at school and is unable to enjoy friends and social activities.
- *Persistent*: The distress and confusion continue for weeks, even months, with little relief. (293)

For Pazit Trujillo, living in Jericho had created a severe identity crisis. When she was in Denver, she had constant conflict with her mother, but everything else in her life was functioning. Living in Jericho changed all of this, but she stubbornly wanted to make things work because it had been her choice to come to live with her father. However, she was miserable. If Pazit had remained in her situation in Jericho, she would have been in danger of an identity disorder needing extensive treatment.

TREATMENT: A SCHOOL GUIDANCE COUNSELOR (TANNA M. GARTSIDE) SPEAKS

Q: If you had been a counselor at this particular school, what could you have done to identify the problems that Pazit was having?

A: Pazit's problems could have been alleviated if she had been registered earlier for school. Her father needed to be more responsible by getting his daughter registered two to three weeks before the start of school. All schools are in a state of confusion the week before school starts and during the first week of school. If Pazit's parents had registered her in early August, the school could have given her an orientation. She could also have been matched with a peer counselor, who would have given her a friendship base. As the counselor, I would have made suggestions on how she could be involved with peers in the community and the school. The research of Erikson [1963] makes it clear that adolescence is a time of identity confusion and subsequent searching. Pipher [1994] suggests that girls will grow into healthy adults when they have love from family and friends, meaningful work, respect, challenges, and physical and psychological safety. Identities should come from talents or interests and not just from popularity or sexuality. Pipher also states that girls need skills for coping with stress, self-nurturing skills, and a sense of purpose and perspective. If there is not a feeling of being connected to something larger than themselves, they feel lost. Anxiety, stress, and depression result and prevent success. For Pazit to make a successful transition from Denver to Jericho, she needed a peer support group as well as a strong family base.

Q: Do you think Mrs. Wells, the school nurse, could have been a good resource?

A: Mrs. Wells was probably the only support Pazit had in the school. If she had passed on some information to the school's guidance department about Pazit's frequent visits, an intervention could have been made. Since Mrs. Wells's daughter had also experienced prejudice in the school, she could have talked to Pazit and helped her. Mrs. Wells was very supportive, but I would have liked to see her refer Pazit to someone else for further action.

Q: What could have happened if the nurse had taken action?

A: Pazit may have been given some help with coping skills. As a counselor, I felt that Pazit took the easy way out by leaving Jericho High School. I realize that she had experienced extreme harassment and even persecution. But challenges help people grow, and experience can be the best teacher. If Pazit had stayed at Jericho and worked through the problems, she would have been a stronger adult. With assistance from school personnel and at least one or two friends, she could have made it. Pazit's presence in the school could have been a learning experience for Jericho High's student body. We live in a multicultural society where people must learn to live with one another.

Q: How would you have been able to smooth the way for Pazit in her relationship with the town members?

A: I would have found some girls in that school who were brave enough to become her friends. I would have asked a teacher who lived in the community to work with her in the transition. In the 1950s my family moved from a northern community to a very rural southern town. There was still prejudice toward "Yankees." I came from a wealthy, progressive school district with a large secondary school of one thousand students, to a K-12 school with two hundred students; only twenty-seven were in my class. There was ample opportunity for harassment and prejudice. My parents and teachers were very supportive. Instead of being an outcast, I graduated as student government president and valedictorian of my class. Pazit's personality may have set her up for failure. She may have had an unrealistic vision of who she was. She needed to give a little; to try to fit in without compromising her values.

Q: What about the parents? Could you have spoken to them about Pazit's situation?

A: Girls need loving and supportive parents. The parents should have been called in for a conference, or a home visit should have been made. But at the beginning of the school year, the staff is swamped with details. If there was not a system in place for follow-up with new students, I may not have been aware of the seriousness of the problem. Again, Pazit needed to seek out help from the resources available in her school. She needed to show some trust toward those in a position to help her.

Q: Is there anything you could have done about the actions of Mr. Dalrymple, the bandleader? I don't care what kind of a school it is: The faculty certainly has a responsibility to be open minded. Why wasn't it suggested to him early on that he compromise his original plans for the marching formation because of Pazit's visible discomfort with those plans?

A: This is another place the counselor could have been involved. Obviously, Pazit was not out to destroy the band, although the bandleader certainly felt threatened by her. He could, of course, have handled the situation better. And that is one of the responsibilities of the school counselor—to help when situations arise between school personnel and the students. But the counselor cannot help if she or he is not aware of the problem. With a proper orientation to the school, Pazit would have known that the guidance counselor was a resource to help if there was a problem with a teacher.

Q: What would you have done in this situation?

A: In many high schools there is a counselor assigned to ninth graders to focus on their special transitional needs. This counselor would have made time to take an interest in, concentrate on, and help that child. Since Pazit did not attend the summer band camp, the obvious step would have been to try to find someone else who was new to town and also registered in the band. A successful strategy for me as a counselor has been matching up new students so they can be "buddies" to each other. In at least one such situation, the "buddies" ended up being very close friends.

Q: Suppose you had known about the bandleader's actions: the in-class prayers, the cross formation, etc. What would you have done?

A: Schools have their own political structure. With a very successful bandleader, it may be hard for a counselor to intervene effectively. The bandleader felt he was right in what he was doing. He had the support of parents and a history of success. If there were a professional relationship of respect and trust built between the counselor and the bandleader, some intervention may have been made. The critical issue was Pazit playing from the sidelines. She was setting herself up for ridicule by the whole band when she was visibly playing in that position. If there were a positive relationship with Mr. Dalrymple, I would have suggested an alternative plan giving her a special responsibility, but not in the formation. If there were not a good relationship, it is probable that I would not want to say anything. It appeared throughout the story that Mr. Dalrymple was more interested in winning awards than helping students. But, in his defense, a successful, award-winning band program would bring college scholarships to his students. So, in his eyes, he was helping his students.

Q: Another major influence upon the children's thinking were the weekly church youth group meetings. Could you have spoken there?

A: I doubt that I would have been involved there, in talking to the leader about his group. Judging by Brother Kent Secrist's comment in response to Billy's question about the Jews, "Well, sure, we want to bring Jews to the Lord Jesus" [111], it is doubtful that the church would have been open to helping Pazit feel more at home in the community. The only hope might have been the study of world religions in school. Diversity and multicultural understanding are being incorporated into various curricula. Florida requires the study of the Holocaust. Jericho High School needed to make some changes in the curriculum to meet the needs of the changing student body. *The Diary of Anne Frank* is typically required reading for eighth graders, so at this point the students should have had some exposure to diversity in religion. I would have hoped that the students in that community would have shown curiosity, or even just tolerance, rather than exhibit the fear they did. But peer pressure (and parental approval) are powerful things to adolescents, and, judging by the way Pazit's objections to Mr. Dalrymple's plans were made public, Pazit—and therefore her religion—were made to seem a threat. Billy himself thought the band director to be the second most important person in the school, and maybe the entire town. Mr. Dalrymple brought the trophies home to the town.

Q: What did you think about Pazit's father's actions?

A: Of course he overreacted. He failed to take her feelings into consideration, as his first mistake, and then he acted so as to turn the responsibility over to someone else. In fact, he was kind of a manipulator; he sat back and watched. He didn't handle the situation well at all. Most schools actively seek parental involvement (naturally, they prefer that support to tell them what they are doing right). Pazit's father needed to talk to the school personnel himself. I think Mr. Trujillo would not have considered legal action if he thought the school was making some attempt to respond to his daughter's needs. Once the ACLU became involved, the battle lines were drawn.

Q: What about Pazit's natural mother's role, back in Denver? Although she does try to involve herself in Pazit's life, calling on the telephone and doing a fair amount of worrying, she obviously has her own high expectations for her daughter and is consequently a little out of touch with her daughter's needs. Do her expectations have anything to do with this story?

A: Her mother expected Pazit to make good grades, she wanted to talk to Pazit's father when she found out that Pazit wasn't registered for school, and she telephoned weekly. However, the fights over Leon, a 25-year-old in whom Pazit had been interested at the kibbutz in Israel, Pazit's unsatisfactory grades, and her not living up to her potential created an intolerable relationship between mother and daughter. Ruth, the mother, needed to read Mary Pipher's [1994] book so that she could understand that daughters provoke arguments as a way of connecting and distancing at the same time. I feel Ruth needed to work through the problems with her daughter. They needed to attend at least several sessions with a counselor. Ruth was locked into her own thing, her own expectations, urging Pazit to get into the good classes and so forth, rather than thinking about Pazit's possible difficulties in being new at the school. The mother wasn't communicating with her child and didn't seem concerned with her feelings. Religion and good grades were the most important things to her, not things that might have been more real to Pazit.

Q: How could you have helped in that situation?

A: Not in any way—she was in another town and state. I probably would not have been aware that I should be involved. In middle school, it is not uncommon for parents to call the guidance department and discuss their child's adjustment when there is a change in custody. But by high school it is unlikely that the parent would take the time to do this. It would have been helpful for Pazit if her mother had taken the time to call.

Q: Pazit believed that she could make friends anywhere.

What do you think happened to make her unable to do so at the new school? Should she have, at any time, compromised her feelings, for example, and gone ahead and marched with the band while they did their cross formation?

A: No—her beliefs were too strong. There is a lot of history that might have made it distasteful for her to do that. Not only the religious differences, but the history of persecution of Jews, have made it so.

Q: What might you have done if you could have had all of the book's characters together in one room?

A: The obvious mediation would be between Pazit and the bandleader. He pretended to give in to Pazit by saying that she could play her flute on the sidelines. Maybe he thought he was offering her a compromise, but actually he set her up for persecution.

Q: What compromises might you have suggested to avoid the crisis?

A: The cross formation could have been done more discreetly, for example, if it had to be done at all, by putting it at the very end and creating another role for Pazit so that she participated as a player in everything but the last piece, then assumed a new responsibility.

Q: How could you have suggested that?

A: We could have brainstormed some accommodations, some modifications, for this. If I were doing this in a room with them I would ask, "If some students say ugly things to you, what will you do?" I would do this mainly so that the bandleader could get some idea of what Pazit must have been going through and what she was feeling. He could also, through that, get a sense of how something like this might escalate. He's not really selfish—he just can't see beyond what he thinks he's doing for the good of the band and the town.

Q: Would you have called the school staff together?

A: Yes. The administration was not being responsible in this matter. We are living in a different world. We do not realize that if a community is so strong in one way, then they don't have to react. The community took the position that things have been going on this way for a long time without problems, and now there is a problem. Therefore, Pazit herself must be the problem.

Q: What was the real problem here?

A: The religious beliefs in the community were so strong, and they were diametrically opposed to those of Pazit. For instance, a Protestant fundamentalist view of sin would be that all people are born sinful—all humankind is sinful—until they have accepted Jesus. So Pazit is not just different; she is a sinful, bad person because she has not accepted Christ, according to this view. Now, the ACLU got involved because of civil rights and the issue of the cross. Actually, I don't know how the school personnel got away with that in the first place, except that the school board must have all shared those fundamentalist beliefs. The parents advocated it, and the school personnel went along with it.

Q: The author makes reference to the fact that marching in a cross while playing Christian music is illegal in our public schools. Why do you think the school personnel and all of the parents seemed ignorant of that fact?

A: Ellen Scanlon, at the parents' meeting, spoke up for her stepdaughter, Pazit. At that point, a few more adults came forward to say something about freedom of religion and freedom of speech. So they were aware of it. It just hadn't become an issue prior to this because they all shared similar religious beliefs.

Q: Billy also spoke up at that meeting, surprising—and alienating—everyone, including his parents. What was your reaction to that?

A: I wanted to compliment him for speaking up when everybody else was on the other side. At that point he really needed a counselor to talk to because he had set himself up. I'd want the counselor to tell him, "Good for you! You were able to express your opinion in a crowd who you knew was opposed to what you had to say. You stood up for what you believed, even when your family disagreed with you and criticized you." Billy risked a lot that evening, and eventually he was sent to live with an aunt and uncle. He could still benefit by having a counselor or someone to talk to. He needs some help with clarifying whether he really wants to continue the path he has begun heading down. I would ask him what he thought was going to happen as a result of what he had done. I might say, "I personally respect you for expressing your feelings, and for stating your opinion, but what do you think will happen now? What is going to happen to your personal needs as a result of the action that you have taken?" I would keep coming back at him, again and again: "What's going to happen at home? What about your relationship with your mom, dad, and sister? Your girlfriend? Your customers whose lawns you keep mowed and trimmed?" I would not tell him what I think will happen, but instead ask him to think. I would ask, "Are you acting impulsively, or do you know what the consequences will be?"

Q: With regard to Billy's feelings, do we know what prompted the sudden loyalty to Pazit at the risk of the wrath of the community?

A: We really don't know what came first: whether he's just broad minded and open to someone who's different (it was stated that he was initially intrigued by her apparent differences when he first ran into her), or whether his reaction is purely a hormonal, sexual reaction. It could well be an impulsive action, not thought out as to the long-term result.

Q: Suppose you had Pazit in your office right now, in the new community. What would you like to accomplish?

A: I would first ask her, "Are you happy here?"

Q: Do you think she would be honest with you?

A: If I'd established a rapport with her. If the nurse, Mrs. Wells, had opened up the communication, then I don't know. I feel, though, that she would be honest. I'd like to ask her, "What would make you happy here at Jericho High?" and "What are some things that I can do to help you with this transition?" We don't know for sure that she would open up, because of her fears about her father's tendency to overreact. There is also the control factor here; the adolescent wants the freedom to solve his or her own problems without outside help.

Q: What experience have you had in the area of conflict resolution?

A: I brought a conflict resolution program into our school. I brought it in through the back door, starting with some mediation procedures, then I helped it evolve so that the whole school gradually became aware of it. Actually, I was idealistic; I wanted it everywhere. The teachers began to bring it into their curriculum. It's fairly easy to incorporate diversity and conflict resolution issues into the curriculum, especially in the areas of literature and social studies. However, this is such a long-term process, and it's still not where I would like it to be. This is an ongoing project, and results will be visible in time. Even now, however, the results are discernible. We definitely have fewer fights at school, and peer mediation is constantly going on. We've just done a study of students' attitudes toward diversity—whether they believe it's good or bad. In response, students tell us that they feel there is diversity in the school, but I know there isn't that much, really. As a counselor in Pazit's school, I would have approached the director of curriculum and asked how we might incorporate diversity and conflict resolution into the curriculum, how we might integrate it. I would have approached that person who has influence over curricular studies to find out exactly what the school was doing to address issues such as diversity, conflict resolution, student/peer mediation, the Holocaust, etc. I would find these things out.

Q: How did you feel when you finished the book?

A: The ending was kind of convenient. I'm wondering: If Pazit had come to me and asked if I thought she should return to Denver, what would I have advised? Glasser [1965], consistent with the practice of reality therapy that he developed, said to focus on the present and help people understand that all of the actions they choose are their attempts to fulfill their basic needs. I would advise Pazit that if she were trying to decide whether or not to go home for the Jewish High Holy Days, she would just have to lay out the pros and cons and decide which issues were most important to her. I would help her prioritize by adding that if she stayed in the new town, she would get her schoolwork done and would stay in the band; that if she went home, she would get to see her mother and friends, and she would be able to celebrate the holiday. From there she would have to decide which was more important. I might say, "From talking to you, it sounds like you're saying that school is important and band is important. If you go home, you'll get behind at school, but then you can see your mom and communicate with her and celebrate the holidays with people of your own faith. What is more important to you?"

STUDENTS' REACTIONS TO *DRUMMERS OF JERICHO*

We asked 15-year-old Mary Paiva and Brett Dean, also 15, to read the book, and we met with them to discuss their reactions. Mary and

Brett had some interesting insights to offer us, and we found their perspectives enlightening.

Q: Brett has already said that he liked the book. What did you think, Mary?

M: I found it very interesting. It was realistic even though it was disappointing, but I felt that was probably what would happen. A lot of times, people discriminate. At this point it really is the truth. It is what would happen.

Q: Were you able to relate to Pazit?

M: Well, I guess in a way, because so many of my friends are Christian, although they're many different denominations. As much as they're Christian, they do live it. If you live the life of a Christian, it's a stigma, but if you don't, it's also a stigma.

Q: Were you able to relate to anybody else in the book?

M: Billy's sister, the cheerleader. I reacted to her in a negative way. The cheerleaders were very conceited. That was my first opinion of them, that they were conceited.

Q: How did you feel about Pazit's relationship with her parents?

M: Her natural mother seemed to be pushing her about the grades. I think part of the reason for Pazit's leaving was a form of rebellion, a way to get back at her mother. My own mother was actually a good influence when I started having trouble with my grades at one point. She was very supportive and never yelled or anything.

Q: How did she help you when things got bad?

M: She gave encouragement. Sometimes she even sat down while I was completing homework assignments and did her work, sitting next to me. There was the feeling that someone cared. That's what Pazit needed and what she wanted Billy to become for her: her rock to hold on to for support.

Q: Why do you think Pazit avoided talking to her natural mother about her problems at the new school?

M: There was such a lack of communication between them. In addition, she had left her mother for her father, against her mother's wishes, so she had to make it sound as if things were going well. She couldn't let her mother say, "I told you so."

Q: What did you think about her stepparents? Did they take enough responsibility?

B: I'm still trying to decide whether the stepfather overreacted in bringing in the ACLU. Pazit didn't have any problem standing on the sidelines, but *he* did. However, I think he did the best that he knew how.

M: I was very happy with the stepmother because she went beyond what she had to do. Pazit wasn't even her daughter, but she crossed the line into motherhood. She made a lot of compromises and was willing to make concessions.

Q: What if you'd been in Pazit's school? What would you be going through?

M: There are always friends. My first reaction was that she needed a real friend. I switched schools between elementary and middle school, and it was hard to get to know my new schoolmates. In three years I ended up with only a few good friends. It takes a long time for me to call them friends.

Q: Another thing we want to ask you about is the relationship between Mrs. Wells and Pazit.

B: That was nice. I liked the fact that the nurse supported her.

M: I can relate to this, too. I had a teacher like Mrs. Wells. When I had a verbal fight at school, it hurt. So I went down to the office, and there was Mrs. P. She was like a second mother, just because of her nature, so this seemed to be a realistic situation.

Q: What did you think about Billy's actions?

B: I can understand him going against his family's opinion. He came through for Pazit, in the end.

Q: What would you say to Billy about his actions?

B: I would tell him that he did a good thing. That it's really hard to stand up against someone. I don't know if I could do that. He's got a lot of strength.

Q: What about the fact that he left the school and went to live with his uncle?

B: That was best. If he'd stayed, there might have been trouble.

Q: So you feel like the townspeople wouldn't have forgiven him?

B: Over a long time. But even if they forgave him, it might never be forgotten. He'd always be the guy who messed up the marching band.

Q: What were your feeling about Billy's parents?

B: That was a problem because they had their own ideals for him. Each of them did: his father, mother, brother, and sister.

M: They put unrealistic pressures on him to be popular, rather than letting him just fit in. They wanted him to be more. They made comments that he would lower the family's reputation, and they were worried about how his actions made them look.

B: His mother said, "How can you do that to me?" She didn't ask, "What were you feeling?" or, "Are you all right?"

Q: Suppose you were in a position to know Pazit. What kinds of conversations might you have had with her?

M: I had a Jewish friend in the fifth-grade whose grandmother owned a bookstore. We weren't really talking much about religion at that age; it was more about books. But I understand why Pazit refused to march. Although my own religion is based on the Jewish faith, I would still be against marching in a Star of David, so I can relate to Pazit's not wishing to march.

Q: Do you think you could have found common ground with Pazit?

M: I'm very much in touch with my Christian beliefs. However, my fifth-grade friend and I became such good friends that religion didn't really matter. That would probably happen again.

Q: At school, did you ever have any situations comparable to the ones described in the book?

M: I was one of five new students because of the transition into the middle school. Although there were five of us, there was still an awkward stage before I found my niche. I believe every teen goes through a similar stage.

Q: I was going to ask you if you'd experienced any discrimination. At times I felt that maybe Pazit did not do enough to relate to her peers, that maybe she was putting up a wall there.

M: I wouldn't blame her. Maybe she was more frightened than she let on, and that's why she put up that barrier.

Q: I hear you saying that maybe the student body had more of a responsibility to reach out and help her.

B: I think she should have been more open. What I did do, and try to do still, is jump in and talk to new people. And she could have been a little more open and try harder to make friends. Actually most of the student body didn't like her, not because she was Jewish, but because she made problems with the band.

Q: The first day at school, she walked in and no one acknowledged her existence. No one would eat with her. The student body just pushed her away. How do you think that might have affected her? I have a feeling that her distinctive style of dress was a major issue. I always tell new kids when they're coming for orientation that there are some things they might want to wear or not wear.

M: I kind of feel that she came in with an open mind.

Q: The thrust that schools today have in terms of teaching about diversity is very strong. We are addressing the issue of multiculturalism in the schools. Do you think that it's had a positive effect?

M: Well, because of that, you can accept differences now. But you still have to have common ground when you make friends with someone. It's not a stigma if you're white and you have a black friend, for example. Initially, you have to have common interests, though, and then later your friendship is strengthened by your shared memories.

Q: I do see more friendships among adolescents who do not share the same cultural or racial background. But because so many people in this country, from the vast majority of cultural backgrounds, are Christian, I wonder if that might not be a common factor for them. Might there be more of a disparity when religion is not shared?

M: Yes, because that wouldn't be a common interest on which to start a friendship. But they should have looked beyond that, for something else.

Q: What about the other teachers? How do you feel about their reactions when Pazit indicated to them that she was having problems?

M: The only time she tried to talk was toward the end. The teachers said that the principal had told all the teachers not to talk about it. Also, she's just another student. There can be quite a distance between students and teachers. There are only one or two students who stand out each year above the rest.

Q: Do you think that's a real problem?

M: Teachers have hundreds of students. Once you start changing classes, then it's very hard. This year when I was homeschooled, I visited my mom's classroom, and I actually learned the names of all thirty-five children right away. But this was only one class. If there were more than one—if I don't even know the students who are my peers—then how could a teacher be expected to know every student?

Q: Have you stopped to think that the whole story took place in just a little over a month? Did you think maybe Pazit didn't give it a good try? Did she throw in the towel too quickly? I'm a little annoyed—her reaction seemed to be to flee whenever anything went wrong. She left her mother for Israel, left her mother again for her father, and then left her new school to return to her mother.

M: Some people are too afraid of the unknown. They don't want to think about their options: what will happen if they stay, what will happen if they go. She ran away instead of dealing with her problems.

Q: Was there someone who might have helped her better deal with her problems, someone to talk to so that she might not have had to run away?

M: This is something she's going to have to work out for herself. There are plenty of people to help you and realize that your problem is there, but that's all they can do. It's up to you to change your own personality. [Mary's comment illustrates the control factor that many adolescents experience.]

Q: We have felt that there is a lot in this book about dealing with identity crises. Do you know what we mean when we talk about a young person's identity crisis?

M: Yes, it's who, what, where do you want to be? Where do you fit in? What crowd do you want to be in?

Q: Yes. The big issue, encompassing her parents' divorce, her former friendships and relationships, and the prejudice she encountered, was that Pazit was trying to figure out who she was. Do you think she came to any culmination of that? Did this situation help, or hurt, Pazit in finding out who she was?

M: It helped her feel stronger. She ended up knowing what it was she believed. It will take her a long time to get over it, though. It hurt her.

B: It hurt Billy, too, though.

M: Yes, she dragged him down. The price of her gaining her identity was the loss of his. Now he has to decide who he is, what he stands for, and where he is in the world. It's a leapfrog effect: One jumps over another, who is then behind, and so on.

Q: What kind of effect do you think that had on Billy?

M: It made him independent. Before meeting her, he was satisfied just to fit in. Now he's an independent person who isn't afraid to express his own views. Throughout the book I kept asking, "Why?" So many events brought this question up. I asked myself, "Why did this have to happen?" or, "Why can't we all get along?"

The most important point to come out of our meeting with the two students was that Pazit made strides in discovering her identity at Billy's expense. Mary and Brett seemed to accept as normal the fact that Pazit's leap in growth was acquired through the downfall of another. In this case, Billy lost, whether or not temporarily, his friends, family, community, band—*everything* he had.

RECOMMENDED READINGS

Fiction

Arrick, Fran. (1981). *Chernowitz!* New York: Penguin. 183 pp. (ISBN: 0–451–16253–6). MS, HS.

Bobby Cherno, a ninth grader, is secure in his identity and popular with his friends until he meets up with a bully named Emmett. Emmett's tormenting escalates into a campaign of hatred and prejudice against Bobby, who must decide whether to allow the persecution or to fight back.

Blume, Judy. (1970). *Are You There God? It's Me, Margaret.* New York: Dell. 149 pp. (ISBN: 0–440–90419–6). ES, MS.

Eleven-year-old Margaret talks to God daily, but with one of her parents Christian and the other Jewish, she is confused about which God she is talking to. Her concerns about fitting in are reflected by her indecision as to whether she should join the YWCA or the Jewish Community Center. When a teacher requires a year-long project, Margaret chooses to research religion.

Clifford, Eth. (1985). *The Remembering Box.* Boston: Houghton Mifflin. 70 pp. (ISBN: 0–395–38476–1). ES, MS.

Nine-year-old Joshua learns about his Jewish heritage and the importance of family tradition through his grandmother's stories and her box of keepsakes.

Cormier, Robert. (1992). *Other Bells for Us to Ring*. New York: Dell. 144 pp. (ISBN: 0–44–040717–6). MS.

When Darcy, whose family is Protestant, moves into a Catholic neighborhood, she overcomes her feelings of isolation through her new friendship. She learns about differences in religious practices and beliefs, and her understanding helps her through the great loss she suffers.

Crew, Linda. (1989). *Children of the River*. New York: Dell. 213 pp. (ISBN: 0–440–21022–4). MS, HS.

While a young teen, Sundara is forced to flee her native Cambodia. As she begins a new life in America, her adolescence is made more difficult by being caught between two conflicting cultures. But when she is befriended by an American boy, despite their classmates' open prejudice, Sundara learns to bridge the gap between her past experiences and the opportunities she now sees before her.

Farmer, Nancy. (1993). *Do You Know Me?* New York: Orchard. 105 pp. (ISBN: 0–531–05474–8). ES.

Tapiwa's uncle Zeka brings new experiences to Tapiwa in Zimbabwe and provides a different kind of education from what she is receiving at the Lobatse School. Her haughty classmates shun her because she is poor and resent her because she is so intelligent. Eventually, she is removed from the school.

Fine, Anne. (1997). *The Tulip Touch*. Boston: Little, Brown. 149 pp. (ISBN: 0–316–28325–8). MS.

When Natalie moves to a new community, she becomes attracted to Tulip, who is ostracized by her peers. The friendship is marred by Tulip's menacing and dangerous behavior, but Natalie feels she's under a spell and can't get out. Eventually, Natalie summons her inner strength and learns that she doesn't always have to tacitly accept others' actions.

Garrigue, Sheila. (1985). *The Eternal Spring of Mr. Ito*. New York: Aladdin. 163 pp. (ISBN: 0–689–71809–8). MS, HS.

To Sara, England in the early 1940s seemed like a different world. Now that she's been evacuated to Vancouver, life is peaceful and calm. But when the Japanese bomb Pearl Harbor, Sara's safe world is destroyed. Overnight, Mr. Ito, her uncle's gentle Japanese gardener, has become the enemy. Sara must defy her family in order to continue her friendship with Mr. Ito and his family.

George, Jean Craighead. (1994). *Julie*. New York: HarperCollins. 226 pp. (ISBN: 0–06–023528–4). MS, HS.

A coming-of-age novel, this sequel to the Newbery Award–winning *Julie of the Wolves* chronicles Julie's transition between two worlds. She must identify which values are important to her as she struggles to make sense of the conflicts between her traditional Inuit heritage and the modern world.

Greene, Bette. (1993). *Summer of My German Soldier*. New York: Dell. 208 pp. (ISBN: 0–44–021892–6). MS, HS.

Sheltering an escaped German prisoner of war is the beginning of some shattering experiences for a 12-year-old Jewish girl in Arkansas. Patty Berger sees the escapee not as a Nazi soldier, but as a lonely, frightened young man with feelings not unlike her own. While patriotic feelings run high in the community, Patty risks losing family, friends, and even her freedom for this dangerous friendship.

Nonfiction

Caron, Ann F. (1991). *Don't Stop Loving Me: A Reassuring Guide for Mothers of Adolescent Daughters*. New York: HarperCollins. 228 pp. (ISBN: 0–06–097402–8). A.

Based on interviews with many adolescent girls and their mothers, this book guides mothers in their effort to facilitate their daughters' easy passage into adulthood, with a common-sense approach. Issues include physical and emotional changes in the adolescent.

Douglas, Susan J. (1995). *Where the Girls Are: Growing Up Female with the Mass Media*. New York: Random House. 340 pp. (ISBN: 0–8129–2530–0). MS, HS, A.

TV sitcoms, records, magazines, and movies will form, for better or for worse, the culture that girls will share with other people.

Eagle, Carol J., and Carol Colman. (1994). *All That She Can Be: Helping Your Daughter Achieve Her Full Potential and Maintain Her Self-Esteem during the Critical Years of Adolescence*. New York: Simon & Schuster. 288 pp. (ISBN: 0–671–88554–5). MS, HS, A.

Girls 14 to 16 enter a highly experimental period in which they "try on" many different roles. The middle-adolescent girl opens herself up to a world of possibilities. She daydreams about the kind of woman she wants to become, and she seeks a positive identity while flirting with many potential careers and lifestyles.

Elkind, David. (1984). *All Grown Up and No Place to Go: Teenagers in Crisis*. Reading, MA: Addison-Wesley. 232 pp. (ISBN: 0–201–11379–1). A.

Dr. Elkind has spent twenty-five years researching and working with teenagers in crisis. Issues covered in this book include family and peer relationships, cultural influences, and the effects of stress. Parents, counselors, and teachers will find this book useful.

Hoose, Phillip. (1993). *It's Our World, Too!: Stories of Young People Who Are Making a Difference*. Boston: Little, Brown. 165 pp. (ISBN: 0–316–37241–2). MS, HS, A.

A collection of stories about young Americans who have confronted and conquered injustice by taking a stand for issues they believe in are presented here.

Kaplan, Jeffrey S. (1994). "Using Novels about Contemporary Judaism to Help Adolescents Understand Issues in Cultural Diversity." *School Counselor* 41 (March): 287–295. MS, HS, A.

Dr. Kaplan discusses contemporary novels that may help many adolescents understand how they fit into American society.

Krementz, Jill. (1984). *How It Feels When Parents Divorce*. New York: Knopf. 128 pp. (ISBN: 0–394–75855–2). MS, HS, A.

Nineteen children, age 7 to 16, share their stories about what it means to live in a family where divorce occurs, because they want to help other children cope with crises. In many ways, the stories may also help parents understand how they can reduce their children's angst during difficult times.

Minuchin, Salvador. (1984). *Family Kaleidoscope*. Cambridge, MA: Harvard University Press. 246 pp. (ISBN: 0–674–29231–6). HS, A.

Dr. Minuchin, a well-respected family therapist, explores issues with adolescents and their families. He presents interviews and anecdotal data about divorce, stepfamilies, and transitioning, among other topics.

REFERENCES

Erikson, Erik. (1963). *Youth: Change and Challenge*. New York: Basic Books.
Erikson, Erik. (Ed.). (1965). *The Challenge of Youth*. New York: Anchor.
Glasser, William. (1965). *Reality Therapy: A New Approach to Psychiatry*. New York: Harper & Row.
Kaplan, Jeffrey S. (1993). "Merry Christmas Jeffrey Kaplan: A Review of Adolescent Novels about Contemporary Judaism." *ALAN Review* 21 (fall): 1–6.
Kaplan, Jeffrey S. (1994). "Using Novels about Contemporary Judaism to Help Adolescents Understand Issues in Cultural Diversity." *School Counselor* 41 (March): 287–295.
Kaywell, Joan. (1993). *Adolescents at Risk: A Guide to Fiction and Nonfiction for Young Adults, Parents, and Professionals*. Westport, CT: Greenwood.
Meltzer, Milton. (1994). "The Jewish Experience in Multicultural Curriculum." *ALAN Review* 22 (fall): 70–73.
Meyer, Carolyn. (1995). *Drummers of Jericho*. San Diego: Harcourt Brace.
Pipher, M. B. (1994). *Reviving Ophelia: Saving the Selves of Adolescent Girls*. New York: Putnam.
Shaw, Dara Gay. (1995). "The Treatment of Religion and the Independent Investigation of Spiritual Truth in Fiction for Adolescents." *ALAN Review* 22 (winter): 20–22.
Steinberg, Laurence, and Ann Levine. (1990). *You and Your Adolescent*. New York: Harper & Row.
Teasley, Alan B., and Ann Wilder. (1994). "Teaching for Visual Literacy: Fifty Great Young Adult Films." *ALAN Review* 21 (spring): 18–23.

CHAPTER 10

Identity from Destructive Behavior: Robert Cormier's *Tunes for Bears to Dance To*

Janet E. Kaufman and Lynn Kaufman

In *Tunes for Bears to Dance To*, Robert Cormier presents us with an 11-year-old boy who eventually feels himself coerced into destructive, violent behavior. Henry—a curious, grieving, seemingly gentle, working-class boy—destroys the artwork, the memory work, of Mr. Levine, a Holocaust survivor who has been a model of creativity and courage. Although Henry commits this act, we know from Cormier that the older man and the young boy had felt compassion for each other. The questions about human behavior and human responses that the book raises do not differ dramatically from the questions that writers, thinkers, and reflective people have asked about the Holocaust and other extreme situations of the twentieth century.

SYNOPSIS

On the very first page of the novel, we meet Henry, the protagonist, who is describing a "crazy house." Of all the comings and goings on his street, the "crazy house" and the old man going to and from the "crazy house" are what catch Henry's eye and capture his imagination. His mother corrects his language, telling him that "it's an institution for the insane" (2). However, the fact that it is known as a "crazy house" poses a question for Henry as he next describes the old man, Mr. Levine, who walks out of that house each morning. "He does not look either crazy or insane," but actually "normal" (2). Henry notices that by afternoon, though, when the old man returns, he looks "like stone worn away by years of rain" (2). Only later will Henry begin to understand the reasons for Mr. Levine's weariness.

As Henry considers his own state of mind, he seems aware of a continuum of difference between "normal" and "crazy" in himself and others. One phenomenon of adolescence, as Kohlberg and Gilligan have understood it, is "the discovery of the subjective self and of subjective experience as something unique" (Appleyard, 1991, p. 96). Adolescents begin experiencing themselves as divided between an inner self, which is the locus of unique feelings, opinions, and thoughts, and an outer self, which plays roles and puts on appearances for others. Furthermore, as adolescents' ability to think abstractly about the world develops, they concurrently gain the ability, as Appleyard says, "to think about thinking, to reflect critically about [their] own thoughts" (97).

Henry describes himself as being not fully "normal" (2). We learn, however, that Henry had lost his younger brother, Eddie, one year previously, to a hit-and-run accident. Henry worries throughout the novel about himself and his parents, who resemble, like Mr. Levine, "stone worn away by years of rain." Henry briefly considers suicide but realizes that this, in fact, would "bring even more sorrow to his parents" (3). Thus, with the advent of adolescence, as we go on to discover, Henry finds himself worrying about such weighty concerns as life and death, grief and guilt, physical abuse, prejudice, violence, and destruction. Facing problems with—or without—his grieving parents will create the need for him to make immediate decisions and choices with complex ramifications.

Through his after-school jobs as a "bender" (one who bends to stack the shelves with food in the corner grocery), Henry finds himself in an interdependent relationship with the grocery owner, Mr. Hairston, a man who at first seems to be an understanding and consistent adult. Not too far into this relationship, however, Henry gains glimpses into his boss's character. He hears Mr. Hairston call a friend "a grease ball," a Jewish man a "kike," Mr. O'Brien an "Irisher," and Mrs. Karminski a "Polack" (5). However uncomfortable he may feel about Hairston's comments, Henry continues working at the store every day until he breaks his leg and cannot work for several weeks. At this time, he learns more about his boss. "Mr. Hairston scowled at his broken foot, in fact, scowled most of the time. His expression was as sour as the pickle in the wooden barrel" (7). Slowly, Henry realizes that Hairston sees more negative than positive attributes in people. Clearly disliking the labels that Hairston gives to the different people who shop in the store, Henry makes an effort to describe his observations about people as positive and life giving, and, on rare occasion, he speaks back to Hairston. When Hairston calls Mrs. Karminski "dumb" and "a Polack," Henry asserts, "I think she's lonesome. Her husband died last month" (5). But most of the time, Henry keeps quiet—he needs a job.

In his loneliness, Henry's fascination with Mr. Levine grows. He is curious about Levine's "trance" and his "changes of expression"—from apparent contentment to expressions of sadness and grief, to looks of fright when approached by a stranger: Mr. Levine would "lurch back as if expecting a blow" (19). When Henry decides to follow Mr. Levine, he ends up at the door to the arts and crafts center that the old man enters each day. Once inside, Henry witnesses Mr. Levine carving "a miniature village of houses and barns, populated by the wooden figures which represented his family and friends in his youth" (22). Watching Mr. Levine whittle away at the blocks of wood, Henry learns that Mr. Levine's strange language is Yiddish and that his carving represents his effort to revive the family, friends, and village he lost in the Holocaust. Although Henry remembers Mr. Hairston's derogatory comments about Jews, he sustains his interest in Mr. Levine's project, fascinated by Mr. Levine's talent, determination, and commitment to remembering (25).

Meanwhile, Henry remains absorbed in his family's grief and memories, and attempts to help his parents grieve. He accompanies his mother to the cemetery, wondering how he could mark his brother's life at the grave. With his mother, he begins to dream about a monument of a baseball and bat to memorialize and honor Eddie. Observing Henry, Hairston becomes aware of Henry's desire for this monument. Knowing or sensing Henry's desperation and his vulnerability to suggestions from others, Hairston begins leading Henry into a situation that is both tempting and dangerous. He attempts to make a Faustian bargain with Henry: If Henry agrees to covertly destroy Mr. Levine's crafted *shtetl*, his Jewish village, Hairston will reward him with a stone monument for Eddie's grave and a promotion for his mother. Upon Henry's immediate cry of "No" in response, Hairston tells him to think about the bargain before answering so quickly; for if Hairston cannot trust Henry to accomplish this little goal, how can he trust Henry in the store? To this boy who already feels vulnerable and does not understand the degree of power that adults do and do not have over children, Hairston takes on a godlike character here. Henry now needs to learn huge lessons: how to distinguish the power that individuals have and the nature of that power and how to trust himself in the realm of moral choice.

When Hairston asks Henry to commit this violent act—an act Hairston himself is unable or unwilling to commit—he sees an opportunity to coerce Henry into a situation that would steal his innocence, thereby bolstering Hairston's own sense of power through bigotry, violence, and destruction. Hairston's bargain confuses Henry: While Hairston seems to regard Henry with affection, as if Henry were a favorite son, he simultaneously asks Henry to be destructive. Not able to decide whether or not to meet Hairston's demand, Henry sneaks into the arts and crafts center one night as if to test himself. Still not sure what to do, he finds a mallet and raises it above Mr. Levine's village, bringing himself to a ready position for carrying out the terrible deed. Then, at the final moment of decision, a rat leaps out, and Henry, terrified, jumps in reaction, dropping the mallet on the village. When Henry returns from inadvertently destroying the village, Hairston, attempting to bond with Henry through this act and thereby justify his own impulses, winks at the boy, "drawing them into a kind of conspiracy" (92). Hairston alerts him, "You see Henry, you are like the rest of us, after all, not so innocent. Not so innocent, are you?" (94).

GENESIS: THE ARCHETYPE

Cormier gives us a version of an ancient story—the story of human sacrifice. As it evolves, Henry's situation appears strikingly similar to the story of the binding of Isaac in the biblical Book of Genesis, one of the most terrifying, haunting stories in all of literature. In this story, God asks Abraham to bring Isaac to Him as an *olah*, an offering that has been totally consumed. Isaac, we remember, was the son of Abraham's old age, the one he and Sarah had waited for until they were in their nineties. Abraham takes Isaac up Mount Moriah, builds an altar, lays the wood on it, binds Isaac, and lays him on the altar. Then, as Abraham stretches out his hand with the knife to slay his son, an angel of God calls out to Abraham from the heavens and tells Abraham not to touch Isaac; for in the act of binding Isaac, Abraham has already demonstrated his fear of God, and there is no need for the sacrifice itself. At this point, Abraham looks up and sees a ram caught in a thicket, and Abraham sacrifices the ram instead of Isaac.

The basic characters in this story—the figure of God, the compliant servant, Isaac, the sacrifice, and the ram—directly correlate to those in Cormier's story. Hairston (the godlike figure) tries to make a pact, a covenant, with Henry (the servant) that includes rewards for fulfilling the pact. Mr. Levine's village becomes the sacrificial object, and the ram from the Genesis story finds its correlative in the rat that leaps into Henry's sight as he stands on the bench in the arts and crafts center with the mallet above his head, ready to smash the village. Whether or not Cormier meant to make this analogy in his novel, the archetypal quality of his story raises significant questions.

First, how do we choose the leaders we will follow? How do we distinguish between good leaders and dangerous leaders? Hairston appears godlike to Henry, demanding complete trust and seeming to have the power to create and destroy life. How, then, do we develop a sense of self strong enough to recognize when a seemingly good leader becomes threatening? What kind of conditions prepare us or lead us to make the decisions we are called upon to make? Furthermore, when we sacrifice, how do we determine what and whom, exactly, we are giving up? Do we sacrifice ourselves in the act of obedience? Abraham, for instance, in addition to risking the life of his son, risked his relationship with God and even his faith in God. Does a sacrifice test what it means to put oneself on the edge; what it means to be caught at that moment of contemplating destruction; what it means to capitulate, obey, and then discover, as Henry does, that one is not the patriarch Abraham with an angel of God watching over him while he stands on the precipice, but a common person?

We do not propose to answer these questions here. Cormier's book, however, helps us ask the questions. And, as Henry begins to answer them for himself, he teaches his readers about what it means to develop one's own path toward moral conduct, just as our students and clients constantly teach us to see from yet another perspective and to ask our questions in new ways.

SEARCHING FOR IDENTITY

As he interprets the tension between childlike and adult behaviors in adolescence that Erikson describes, Appleyard (1991) stresses that adolescents have "to integrate an identity among the competing impulses of trusting peers and elders who will give imaginative scope to their aspirations, but simultaneously feel they must oppose anyone who sets limits to their self-image and ambition" (98). The adolescent's task becomes one of trying on new behaviors, new attitudes, new relationships—new ways to be in the world. At the moment in his life when we meet Henry, his self-awareness begins to develop through painful lessons, determining the moral identity he will carry into adulthood.

As *Tunes for Bears to Dance To* opens, Henry finds himself in the midst of a family crisis that complicates his own developing identity. His parents, entrenched in grief from the sorrow and pain of the death of their younger son, Eddie, show no sign of recovering and remain emotionally unavailable to Henry. Although his parents had moved after Eddie's death, Henry realizes that they "had not left Eddie behind in Frenchtown, after all" (7). The grief followed them even though "the car that struck Eddie sped away and was never seen again" (8).

Throughout the time period of the novel, Henry feels and witnesses a great deal of anger. He feels angry that his childhood in Frenchtown had come to a startling halt with Eddie's death, and anger and disappointment that his parents had descended into inconsolable grief after the death. He sees his own anger when his friend, Jack Antonelli, taunts him about his father being "crazy" (42) and when he finds out his father has to go to the hospital for the "disease" of sadness (56). At first Henry thinks that anger is better than sadness and pounds his fists on his bed, but then he cries anyway, finding himself caught between competing emotions. In another instance, Henry sees his mother taking out her anger on him and on his father after receiving no tip one day from her waitressing job. In the grocery, he observes the bruised cheek of Hairston's daughter and then becomes suspicious of Hairston's potential for great outbursts of anger. He learns much about anger on a much larger scale when the newsreels he had seen about World War II and Hitler's concentration camps become personalized to him through the story of Mr. Levine. With such intensity of feeling and confusion about how to sort through it, and with no adult guidance, Henry steps down deeper into his relationship with Hairston.

READING THE BOOK WITH ADOLESCENTS IN GROUP THERAPY

As a social worker/therapist with preadolescent and adolescent boys in residential treatment, Lynn conducted several group therapy sessions working with *Tunes for Bears to Dance To*, reading the book aloud to ten seventh and eighth graders over a period of several days. The children, all considered severely "at risk," had been removed from their homes for abuse, neglect, and antisocial behavior. They all had experienced loss, and many had sustained years of failed parenting and foster care before entering residential treatment. By the time these children began the daily group therapy sessions, they had witnessed frightening, dangerous, and life-threatening behavior in themselves, their parents, and other adults responsible for them. They described being forced to drive with a drunk foster parent, forced to have sexual relations with adults and other children, and forced to accept beatings with boards, belts, whips, sticks, and branches of trees. They, in turn, came to be physically and, sometimes, sexually violent. Aggression toward themselves and others had become part of their way of life.

These teens often stole food to survive, to feed themselves and younger siblings. They were threatened with more punishment if they revealed abuse; often, however, they kept the abuse secret to protect themselves in case, as one boy said, "no one would believe us and we would be beaten again." Among its other qualities, Cormier's book portrays the ways in which adults fail children; the children in this group identified with that part of the story quickly.

All the children immediately understood Henry's plight with Hairston. Because they had felt powerless in their own situations to voice their concerns, fears, or suspicions of impending danger, they understood how relationships with adults can become frightening. They were fully aware of the influence and control that adults have over them and how easily they could become coerced into silence. Working with them, one saw the survival skills they had acquired for self-preservation. For instance, the children listening to Henry's story immediately understood the temptation of receiving rewards. They related to Henry's perceived need to take care of his parents; many of these children had become "parentified children," children who feel responsible for nourishing and protecting their parents and siblings, and for protecting their family's feelings with hopes of relieving their anger and depression. The children in the group had made decisions and carried out behaviors for which they were ill prepared. They had been compelled to do deeds the implications of which they had not yet had the opportunity, education, or experience to understand.

The children in group therapy questioned Hairston's motives just as Henry did. From the beginning of the novel, upon hearing Mr. Hairston's bigoted comments, they became immediately suspicious of him, and none of his further threats or demands to Henry surprised the children. When Hairston promises a monument for Eddie's grave and a better job for his mother, the children listening to Henry's dilemma knew that

Henry would have to pay a price in return. By the end of the novel, Henry himself understands the exacting price: "It was me he was after all the time. Not just the old man and the village. He didn't want me to be good anymore" (94). Here Henry strikes the core of his moral growth. When children in treatment realize that the adults in their lives do not model or provide opportunities for them to be good, and instead find ways to justify their own bad behavior through children as Hairston does, the children realize that they must separate from the parents or abusers, that they must accept being on their own and moving in a new direction.

In Lynn's experience of treating children who have lived among antisocial and irresponsible adults, she has found the children to feel alone, abandoned, and isolated in their experiences. Reading the book with them and giving them the chance to know that others have experienced similar trauma enabled them to give voice to their suppressed feelings and find sources of strength in the character's successful struggles. More important is helping them understand that the bad behavior into which they feel coerced is never, as Alice Miller (1991) writes, "for [their] own good." Indeed, Hairston nearly did persuade Henry that destroying Mr. Levine's village was for his own good. Not until the village was already smashed did Henry realize that he could never accept the rewards to make the destruction "for his own good." In *Banished Knowledge*, Miller (1991) asserts, "Many people still have no idea that they are placing dynamite in our world when they abuse their children physically or even 'only' physically. They describe their actions as proper and necessary" (4). In fact, after smashing the village, when Henry says that he does not want Hairston's rewards, Hairston tells him that he has to accept the rewards to make the act complete.

Alice Miller (1991) states that for children to develop a moral conscience, they need to internalize the message that they can still love the adults in their lives while acknowledging and admitting that the adults steered them astray. Distinguishing and clarifying this with Henry would, ideally, constitute a significant part of a therapist's work with Henry. To hear that another 12-year-old boy has the strength to stand up to an abusing adult is life giving for frightened children who have been victims of coercion and maltreatment. Henry's story—his personal history, his moral dilemma, and his reaction and responses to that dilemma—echoed the stories of the lives and dilemmas, the reactions and responses of the children in Lynn's group therapy sessions.

The boys in therapy sat completely still listening to Henry's vacillation about whether or not to accept Hairston's bargain. When, toward the end of the novel, Henry finally resists and stands up for himself, refusing to accept Hairston's promised rewards, they cheered and clapped. When asked why, one responded, "Because Henry is learning to make his own decisions. He doesn't owe Mr. Hairston any more bad behavior." The boys' reaction resonates with an incident Robert Coles (1997) recalls in his book *The Moral Intelligence of Children*, in which an adolescent, after watching the film *A Bronx Tale*, says:

> [W]e got lost in that movie . . . you could feel the pull—once you give in and get connected with those people . . . you're through . . . you've given up something that's more important . . . you're not free . . . you're a prisoner, they own you. You let people buy you off and you lose all respect for yourself. You stand up for what you believe—that way, you can look at yourself in the mirror, and you don't need to run and hide . . . you leave a movie like that and your head is all turned on. (19)

Children who have had crimes committed against them usually find it difficult to explain both the crimes and their feelings. They feel angry and resigned when people in a position to hear their story either do not evoke the story or believe it. Social workers repeatedly hear adolescents say, "Why tell anyone? No one believes me anyway." Professionals are trained to believe children, but the children's own parents, teachers, or other significant adults—the "anyone" referred to above—often do not listen to or believe them. In his collection of essays *From the Kingdom of Memory*, Elie Wiesel (1990) explains the perceived "victory of the executioner" in the Holocaust: "[B]y raising his crimes to a level beyond the imagining and understanding of men, [the executioner] planned to deprive his victims of any hope of sharing their monstrous meaning with others" (118). Then Wiesel recalls the tale of a survivor in which an SS officer tells a young Jew, "One day you will speak of all this, but your story will fall on deaf ears. Some will mock you, others will try to redeem themselves through you. You will cry out to the heavens and they will refuse to listen or to believe" (119). The children in group therapy knew this sentiment exactly. One strength of the therapy is in providing a context in which children can share "their monstrous meaning with others," attest to its reality, and find alternative ways of relating to it, besides through repeating the violence they have learned.

THERAPEUTIC INTERVENTIONS: LYNN KAUFMAN'S RECOMMENDATIONS

Given Henry's history, including the recent death of a younger brother, the family's relocation to a new town, the grief-imposed depression of the parents, and the family's loss of income, we know that his family problems at this time are severe. If Henry were my client, I would recommend individual therapy, group therapy, and family therapy. All three would complement each other yet be beneficial in distinct ways.

To better understand Henry, his family dynamics, and the crisis in the family, in family therapy I would make every effort to interview the family for several sessions and assess different perceptions of the problem. Listening to Henry and his parents, I would discover that they were all suffering in different ways and that, occasionally, Henry considered ending his own life (3). It is well documented that when a teen, like Henry, finds "himself/herself alone, at the mercy of a hostile environment, experiencing the loss of a perceived nurturing life-sustaining object . . . and experiencing himself/herself unable to cope with their environment," they are prone to consider, attempt, and complete a suicide (Steinberg and Levine, 1990, p. 325).

Any suggestion of teenage suicide would require immediate attention and thus, first and foremost, the completion of a suicide assessment. The assessment would be crucial for determining the degree of suicide ideation, intention, and planning, and Henry's perceived goal. I would immediately share the results with the family. Since research has shown that primary causes of teenage depression and suicide stem from the family, it is crucial that the family become aware of the intense feelings that lead to such drastic thoughts and actions by one of its children. Many people in the helping professions tend to be cautious or shy about discussing suicide ideation and plans; however, it is essential to talk about suicide as one would discuss any symptoms of any illness that might manifest itself in such permanent, final, and devastating ways. In extensive family therapy I would hope to help Henry and his parents more effectively communicate their grief and concerns to each other and to establish alternate ways of responding to family problems. Addressing the matter of suicide ideation would be the first and most important step in this process.

Continuing to talk with Henry and his parents, I would learn that Henry feels fearful for his parents' well-being as he observes their pain and confusion. However, while attempting to understand the pain and sorrow from Henry's and the family's perspectives, I also would want to begin assessing Henry's and his family's strengths; identifying these strengths in therapy would enable Henry and his family to draw upon them in their efforts to restore their family life.

STRENGTHS PERSPECTIVE

One can find many apparent and admirable strengths in Henry. In the grocery, Henry shows his understanding of the difference between adults' expression of goodness and underlying ill will in his observation of Hairston. He was amazed Hairston could be polite to customers and then insult them behind their backs. As he responds to environmental cues of distress and inappropriate adult behavior, we see not only his ability to sensitively observe but also his potential to articulate his observations and feelings. Henry does not ignore those in pain; each night he prays for his brother Eddie's soul, for his parents' emergence from their grief, for Doris's safety, and for Mr. Levine. Additionally, Henry is self-conscious about his own behavior. When he frightens Mr. Levine by accident, he becomes saddened. His recognition and awareness of his ability to hurt another person demonstrates his capacity for empathy. Later, with his sustained interest in Mr. Levine's crafting of the *shtetl*, Henry shows curiosity about creative outlets for personal expression and respect for other peoples' dedication to their own projects. Furthermore, he demonstrates his ability to listen and appreciate others as George, the caretaker of the arts and crafts center, recounts the horrors of war and Mr. Levine's losses.

One hopes that Henry's ability to recognize his own strengths in therapy would increase his self-esteem and ultimately give him a sense of self-control. Perceiving his strengths could give him new understanding and beliefs about himself to call upon in determining his behavior. He could come to understand how multiple, confusing forces—grief, isolation, loneliness, powerlessness—have influenced his decision making.

In therapy, I would want to support Henry's grief from the partial destruction of the village, thereby enabling him to continue developing his own conscience. Henry comes from a situation in which mixed messages from adults have made it difficult to know how to make good choices, so in therapy I would hope to provide an accepting environment, giving Henry some freedom to begin examining his own perception of the consequences of his actions. In such an environment, understanding his guilt, sorrow, and confusion could be a catalyst for developing his

own moral strength and identity. Before destroying the village, he anticipates his own guilt and the sorrow he would feel from hurting Mr.
Levine; and, just before the moment of acting, he hesitates, sweats, and
freezes with his arms holding the mallet above his head. Given his hes-
itance and then his regret, helping him recognize his history of sensitivity
to family members and acquaintances certainly could affirm him and his
ability to protect himself from coercion in the future.

One of the first steps for youth in such situations as Henry's involves
understanding the consequences of their actions. The ability to foresee
consequences prevents destructive and injurious actions, and gives one
the capacity to resist coercion. When an adolescent can no longer be
coerced into negative behavior, the therapist or parents will know that
the young person is developing a conscience for moral conduct.

Adolescence may be the best time for moral questioning and development, and it is perhaps for this reason that young adult literature on
the theme of moral decision making abounds. In *The Moral Intelligence
of Children*, Robert Coles (1997) describes the kind of truth that emerges
for adolescents as a "hatching of eggs," a time when the attitudes, troubles, achievements, and difficulties of childhood reemerge in a more
significant way, so that "young men and women hold on to what they
have got and who they have been for dear life, even as they venture into
new and often fearful territory" (153). Thus, matters of right and wrong
become enormously powerful for adolescents. Coles remembers Anna
Freud saying of an adolescent patient that the patient had wanted "an
alliance between us [the adults] and his superego." As adolescents figure
out their own values and moral codes to give themselves some sense of
direction, they seek, as Coles asserts, a "moral companionship from an
adult or two, be the older person a parent, a teacher, a relative, a friend's
kin" (162). Henry, seeming to need and want just such an adult, chooses
the wrong person. If, in therapy, Henry could begin wrestling with the
question, What is morality? and begin to understand morality to be, as
F. Phillip Rice (1990) says in *The Adolescent*, "a question of how one
human being deals with another human being" (329), I would know that
his work had begun.

Henry will still have to reconcile the reality of his family's situation
with external circumstances. All people, of course, face that task. Teens
and adults alike need support to rally their own selves, to acquire self-
esteem, and to validate their own moral codes. For young people from
situations such as Henry's, learning to delineate possibilities for action
and knowing what is valid or true for oneself takes hard work. In this

case, although Henry did not consciously decide to smash Mr. Levine's village, he did let himself reach the point of standing on top of the bench with the mallet, the point at which the destruction became possible. Angry and humiliated for not standing up for his own sense of rightness, and praying to forgive himself as well as Mr. Hairston at the end of the novel, he knows that he scarred himself through this incident. In the moment of the action, however, he could not anticipate the full extent of the emotional consequences or forgo the perceived opportunity to help his parents and honor his family with a monument for his brother.

CONCLUSION

Henry's conflict raises basic questions: Do we go along with others at the cost of our own integrity, or do we risk rejection by those we choose not to follow? Will we risk losing the perceived protection of leaders with questionable motives? Will we have the courage, strength, and commitment to develop a personal moral code?

The response to these questions ultimately contributes to at-risk adolescents' own survival of traumatic circumstances. One student, who read *Tunes for Bears to Dance To* with a group of at-risk teenage girls for a class project, found that, for these girls, Hairston represented "the afflictions of adolescence" and every situation that might attract them and become beyond their control:

> He was every adult who had mistreated power or brandished authority like a sword. He was the principal who didn't listen to both sides before judging and the father who abused his daughter mentally, physically, and sexually. He was the boy who pushed sex or the vial of cocaine, full of promises and threats. He was the manipulative mother or the best girl-friend who always threatened, "If you don't, I'll never . . ." Mr. Hairston stood as the evil force behind every hard situation. (3–4)

Struggling to survive such "evil forces" and hard situations, these girls saw Henry as a survivor and a role model because he found his way out of Hairston's domination. Another student commented, "He made bad choices, I make bad choices. People don't understand why I do things I do. I won't judge Henry 'cause no one knows what he was thinking on the inside." A third student added, "We all survive choices." As we know, though, not all adolescents do survive the choices they make. At the very end of the novel, Henry gives us some idea of how he survived his entanglement with Hairston.

On one particular night after Hairston proposes the bargain, Henry lies awake, recalling the conversation he had with Hairston when first applying for the grocery job: "Mr. Hairston had asked, 'Can you follow orders? Whether you like them or not?' Henry had answered with a resounding 'Yes' " (77). With this exchange, Cormier raises the stakes of the novel. We might say—as we have found adolescents to say—that the novel directly faces the problem of both authoritarian control and peer pressure. At the same time, we cannot help but hear the echoes of Nazi officers on trial after the war who said, in defense of themselves for having killed hundreds or thousands of innocent people, that they were "following orders." If there was a doubt in our minds about the implications of Henry's decision to go along with Hairston, this passage reminds us that following the wrong leader, seeing a human leader as a godlike figure with powers to reward and punish, can lead us to give up our own power of moral decision making and to symbolically become the Nazi. Fearing Hairston, awed by him, and confusing him with a godlike figure, Henry nearly becomes the Nazi in destroying the replica of Mr. Levine's village. His final refusal to Hairston saves him from that.

In her work *Banished Knowledge*, Alice Miller (1991) claims, "Childhood traumas can be healed if one dares to see them, or they can remain unhealed if one is forced to go on ignoring them" (78). Indeed, Henry sees the injury Hairston caused and, by refusing Hairston's final plea, does not ignore it. To "dissolve pain and fear," to heal injuries like Henry's, Miller believes that children need to be able "to accept full truth of the facts." They need help in exposing the roots of the violence against them, thereby making it possible to examine the phenomena of the violence in the generations that came before them (78–79).

Working from this premise would be a focus of individual, family, or group therapy with Henry. Reading *Tunes for Bears to Dance To* in group therapy created a context for raising direct questions about grief, violence, and pressures within the children's families. Discussing these questions enabled the children to become aware of and acknowledge the roles (such as dictator, bully, victim) that they and their family members play. At one point during the reading of the novel, one boy identified Hairston as a dictator. The group developed a working definition of "dictator," and then the therapist (Lynn) asked directly, "Who were dictators in each of your families?" One by one, going around the room, the boys responded: "My mother." "My father." "My uncle." "My older brother." "Everyone in my family." One boy in the group called out to another boy, whom we shall name "Tommy," that he acted like a dictator among the other kids in the unit. When asked directly, they all were able to name an example of Tommy's dictating, after which Tommy responded, "I admit it. I'm not afraid to admit nothin'." Until the children develop awareness of these roles they play, are able to give language to their experience, and gain some understanding about how the roles shift— from family to peer group to society, from one generation to another— they experience no possibility for change and choice in their behavior. One hopes that in therapy, by continuing to tell their stories, to speak about their torments, to find more language to express themselves, and thus to find the clarity and truth of their experience, the children will find opportunity for change and discover that violence is not necessary.

In the closing paragraph of the novel, Henry prays, as always, for his mother and father, for Eddie, for Hairston's daughter, Delores, and for Mr. Levine. But he "did something he had never done before. He prayed for Mr. Hairston . . . 'Forgive him,' he whispered. '*Forgive me too*' " (101). Many of the university students reading the novel argued that Henry's confession to God and his plea for forgiveness at the end of the novel show more building of moral character than would a direct apology to Mr. Levine. By contending with himself and God, they said, Henry leaves himself vulnerable to his own conscience, enabling self-discipline and, ultimately, empathy to develop and grow. Even more, he shows enormous compassion for Hairston by praying for him, as if he understands something akin to Primo Levi's understanding in *The Drowned and the Saved* (1988) that an "infernal system" such as National Socialism "degrades its victims and makes them similar to itself, because it needs both great and small complicities" (68). Henry seems to appreciate how low Hairston must have fallen in order to try to degrade Henry, in order to need something so terrible from him.

Robert Coles (1997) cites the ability to forgive oneself and others as one of the heights of moral conduct (186). To ask forgiveness, as Henry does, suggests acknowledging one's own behavior and complicity in a situation, facing what happened and thereby becoming able to learn from it. When Mr. Levine discovers his smashed village, he believes the "wise guys" down the street did it and then shows his fondness for Henry by giving him a gift: a hand-carved figure that resembles Henry, with a "big smile on the tiny wooden face." In response to this kind and compassionate gesture, Henry hopes to himself that someday he will "be able to look at it and return the smile" (100). When Henry closes the novel by praying, *"Forgive me too,"* he creates the possibility of giving to himself and others, of showing through his own conduct the meaning of having a moral identity.

RECOMMENDED READINGS

Fiction

Bennett, William J. (Ed.). (1993). *The Book of Virtues.* New York: Simon & Schuster. 818 pp. (ISBN: 0–67157–567–8). ES, MS, HS.

A rich collection of classical tales and myths from around the world. The entries are short, perfect for parents and teachers who want to engage young people in discussion about moral questions and provide pleasure.

Garden, Nancy. (1982). *Annie on My Mind.* New York: Farrar, Straus & Giroux. 234 pp. (ISBN: 0–37440–414–3). HS.

A story of two female high school seniors who fall in love with each other and must face institutional prejudice and find the courage and language to stand up for themselves and what is right.

Gibbons, Kaye. (1987). *Ellen Foster.* New York: Vintage. 126 pp. (ISBN: 0–375703–05–5). HS, A.

The story of a southern girl who believes in herself enough to find her way out of her abusive family and who finds allies in a teacher and foster family. A poignant, rich narrative with a rare mix of trauma and humor.

Greene, Bette. (1991). *The Drowning of Stephan Jones.* New York: Bantam. 224 pp. (ISBN: 0–440226–95–3). HS.

A powerful book confronting the severe expression of hatred and intolerance through the story of Carla, who must decide how to interact with her homophobic boyfriend who torments a gay couple.

Kerr, M. E. (1978). *Gentlehands.* New York: HarperTrophy. 183 pp. (ISBN: 0–06447–067–9). MS, HS.

An adolescent boy faces the discovery that his grandfather, distant from the family but offering a safe haven to his grandson, is a former Nazi in hiding.

Klass, David. (1994). *California Blue*. New York: Scholastic. 199 pp. (ISBN: 0–59046–689–5). HS.

A rich, well-crafted story with complex characters, this novel delves into moral issues regarding ecology and environmentalism through the relationship of 17-year-old John, a track runner and explorer in a nearby redwood forest, to his father, Henry, who is dying of leukemia.

Lowry, Lois. (1993). *The Giver*. New York: Bantam Doubleday Dell. 180 pp. (ISBN: 0–44021–907–8). MS, HS.

A compelling and haunting young adult novel, this Newberry winner could be paired with *1984* or *Brave New World*. With his gift of vision, 12-year-old Jonas begins discovering the cracks in his seemingly utopian world. As he does, he challenges us to look at what we value in ourselves and our communities, and to stand up for freedom and choice.

Matas, Carol. (1993). *Daniel's Story*. New York: Scholastic. 131 pp. (ISBN: 0–590–46588–0). ES, MS.

Daniel's family is forced from its home in Frankfurt, Germany, and sent first to the Lodz ghetto and then to Auschwitz. Daniel struggles for survival and finds hope, life, and even love in the midst of despair. This novel was first published in conjunction with an exhibit about children of the Holocaust at the United States Holocaust Memorial Museum in Washington, D.C.

Williams, Laura E. (1996). *Behind the Bedroom Wall*. Minneapolis: Milkweed. 169 pp. (ISBN: 1–57131–606–X). MS, HS, A.

In 1942, 13-year-old Korinna, an active member of the Nazi Youth, discovers that her parents are hiding a Jewish mother and daughter behind her bedroom wall. How does she respond? Where are her loyalties? And what must she learn?

Wolff, Virginia Euwer. (1993). *Make Lemonade*. New York: Scholastic. 200 pp. (ISBN: 0–590–48141–X). MS, HS.

When 14-year-old La Vaughn becomes the baby-sitter for 17-year-old Jolly's two children, both teenagers discover what it means to help each other grow up. The story appears in poem form and reads very quickly, with extraordinary metaphor and voice.

Nonfiction

Begley, Louis. (1991). *Wartime Lies*. New York: Ivy. 181 pp. (ISBN: 0–804109–90–7). HS, A.

An exquisite, elegiac novel about a Jewish boy escaping the concentration camps by hiding and disguising.

Bierman, John. (1996). *Righteous Gentile: The Story of Raoul Wallenberg, Missing Hero of the Holocaust* New York: Penguin. 264 pp. (ISBN: 0–14024–664–9). MS, HS.

As a diplomat, Wallenberg saved thousands of Hungarian Jews from the fate of the Nazi inferno, then disappeared into the Russian prison system and was never heard from again. This book tells the story of a courageous man and a hero.

Bishop, Claire Huchet. (1984). *Twenty and Ten*. New York: Puffin. 76 pp. (ISBN: 0–140–31076–2). ES, MS.

A powerful story about twenty schoolchildren who hide ten Jewish children from the Nazis in Nazi-occupied France during World War II.

Chiland, C., and J. G. Young. (1997). *Children on Violence: The Child in the Family*. Northvale, NJ: Jason Aronson. 232 pp. (ISBN: 1–56821–235–6). HS.

The question driving this book is: How does violence affect children, and how do children become so violent? The book examines violence in societies around the world, explores the vulnerability of violent children, and presents theory and approaches for preventing these children from succumbing to the violence they learn at very young ages.

Coles, Robert. (1989). *The Call of Stories: Teaching and the Moral Imagination*. Boston: Houghton Mifflin. 237 pp. (ISBN: 0–39552–815–1). HS.

A collection of essays about the role of stories in moral education, rooted in the author's own reading and literary and medical experience.

Frank, Anne. (1997). *The Diary of a Young Girl: The Definitive Edition*. New York: Bantam Books. 335 pp. (ISBN: 0–553–57712–3). MS, HS, A.

The most recent edition of this famous diary includes previously excluded entries in which Anne Frank discusses adolescent sexuality, conflicts with her mother, and reflections on being Jewish.

Hillesum, Etty. (1981). *An Interrupted Life: The Diaries of Etty Hillesum, 1941–43*. New York: Pantheon. 276 pp. (ISBN: 0–805–05087–6). HS, A.

An eloquent, passionate writer in her 20s details her life in the concentration camps.

Innocenti, Roberto. (1996). *Rose Blanche*. San Diego: Harcourt Brace. 32 pp. (ISBN: 0–15–200917–5). MS, HS.

A haunting picture book more appropriate, perhaps, for MS age and over than for young children. About a young German girl who finds a way of sneaking bread to children in concentration camps. As *School Library Journal* wrote, this is "an excellent book to use not only to teach about the Holocaust, but also about living a life of ethics, compassion, and honesty."

Klein, Gerda Weissman. (1957, 1995). *All But My Life*. New York: HarperCollins. 261 pp. (ISBN: 0–80901–580–3). MS, HS.

A heart-stopping autobiography of Klein's stolen childhood and survival of the Nazi death camps. Made into an Academy Award–winning documentary.

Spiegelman, Art. (1986). *Maus*. New York: Pantheon. Vol. 1, 159 pp.; Vol. 2, 136 pp. (ISBN: vol. 1, 0–39474–723–2; vol. 2, 0–67972–977–1). MS, HS, A.

Both an oral history of the author-artist's father, who was a survivor of Auschwitz, and an autobiography, this "graphic novel" enables students to talk about an enormous range of complex literary and historical subjects.

REFERENCES

Appleyard, J. A. (1991). *Becoming a Reader: The Experience of Fiction from Childhood to Adulthood*. Boston, MA: Cambridge University Press.

Boal, Augusto. (1992). *Games for Actors and Non-actors*. Trans. Adrian Jackson. London: Routledge.

Browning, Christopher R. (1992). *Ordinary Men*. New York: Harper Perennial.

Coles, Robert. (1997). *The Moral Intelligence of Children*. New York: Random House.

Cormier, Robert. (1992). *Tunes for Bears to Dance To*. New York: Bantam Doubleday Dell.

Elkind, David. (1981). *Children and Adolescents: Interpretive Essays on Jean Piaget*, 3rd ed. New York: Oxford University Press.

Kohlberg, Lawrence, and Carol Gilligan. (1971). "The Adolescent as a Philosopher: The Discovery of the Self in a Postconventional World." *Daedalus* 100: 1051–1086.

Levi, Primo. (Trans.) (1988). *The Drowned and the Saved*. New York: Summit.

Miller, Alice. (1980). *For Your Own Good: Hidden Cruelty in Child-Rearing and the Roots of Violence*. New York: Noonday.

Miller, Alice. (1991). *Banished Knowledge: Facing Childhood Injuries*. New York: Anchor.

Rice, F. Phillip. (1990). *The Adolescent: Development, Relationships, and Culture*. Boston: Allyn & Bacon.

Steinberg, L., and A. Levine. (1990). *You and Your Adolescent*. New York: Harper Perennial.

Wiesel, Elie. (1990). *From the Kingdom of Memory*. New York: Summit.

CHAPTER 11

Identity through Peers: Paul Zindel's *Harry & Hortense at Hormone High*

Michael L. Angelotti and Terry M. Pace

SYNOPSIS AND LITERARY RESPONSE
(Michael L. Angelotti)

Simply put, *Harry & Hortense at Hormone High* is a contemporary young adult novel based on the Greek myth of Icarus and Daedalus. Under this deceptively innocent title, Paul Zindel has written a story about three young people coming to terms with self-identities in quite different ways. Harry Hickey and his best friend, Hortense McCoy, are reporters for the *Bird's Eye Gazette*—the newspaper of the school they have dubbed "Hormone High" because of the outrageous behaviors of its students and school personnel. Their lives change dramatically when Jason Rohr, a charismatic new student who looks to them like a living Greek statue, asks them to write a story about a hero. Jason confides his belief that he is the reincarnation of the Greek demigod Icarus returned to earth "to lead everyone out of the dark labyrinth" (33–34). Hortense, thinking of herself as a psychiatrist, is fascinated by Jason as a psychological case study, while Harry, a budding writer and voracious reader, finds that Jason whets his appetite as a potential fictional character. In fact, the novel is written as Harry's first-person account of Jason's story. Soon, the three grow beyond their self-serving inclinations and become caring friends. Ultimately, Harry and Hortense discover that although Jason's cloak of godliness initially attracts, it is his human vulnerability that draws them close and touches their lives. In the end, this short, tragic, helping relationship with Jason leads Harry and Hortense to a deeper level of self-understanding.

Significant to each of the three main characters is the concept of "hero" and its importance to the lives of the ordinary people of modern society. In classical Greek style, the novel unfolds as a tale of Jason's quest told by Harry, who, in effect, becomes Jason's Homer or, by Jason's inspiration, Euripides reincarnate. Ironically, woven into the fabric of Jason's quest are the quests of Harry and Hortense, who also are in search of self, although not as dramatically as Jason. To some degree, Harry and Hortense come to terms with it, differently, in the very act of giving of themselves to help Jason when it seems the entire world is against him. Harry and Hortense, then, demonstrate that the world is not entirely demonic, that there is some good. This point is also made in a number of small ways: by the teacher who rushes Jason's dog to the veterinarian, by the caring veterinarian who saves the dog's life, by the kindly school secretary, and by Aunt Maureen.

Harry and Hortense visit Jason at his home in a notorious part of town. They are unsettled by its dilapidated condition and the haglike demeanor of Jason's aunt Mo (Maureen). Jason reveals his plan to save the world, convincing Harry and Hortense (who now believe him to be severely schizophrenic) to meet him at the museum. While there, he is overcome with emotion and breaks down before a mural of his "father" Daedalus. Hortense is moved to type his story for him, unaware that Jason plans to tack it on the school bulletin board, signed "Icarus, a god." Dean Niboff, unforgiving monster of the labyrinth, gives Jason a stern warning and orders Harry and Hortense to disassociate themselves from the "troubled boy."

Harry and Hortense illegally peruse Jason's school records and discover that when Jason was 6, his father had murdered his mother, then committed suicide. Jason's life after that had been one of countless sanitariums and schools. Harry and Hortense resolve to do everything possible to help him. They are put to the test immediately as Jason, now a target of administrative surveillance and peer cruelty, is reinstitutionalized for physically resisting Dean Niboff and other school officials who attempted to stop him from passing out handbills demanding that the school provide a meaningful curriculum.

On a return visit to Jason's house to query Aunt Mo about which institution Jason has been committed to, Harry and Hortense discover that Jason has been constructing a winged hang glider in his garage—clear foreshadowing of his imminent doom. Harry, drawing on his substantial knowledge of literature, reveals to Hortense that Jason's actions parallel those of a classical hero on a quest. As such, he poses no danger to Harry and Hortense, but is bound to engage the demon in a climactic struggle that would inevitably lead to Jason's destruction.

Anxious about Jason's well-being, Harry and Hortense sneak onto the grounds of the Sea Vista Sanitarium for the Young on Staten Island. Whatever remnants of subtle connections to the heroic quest that still exist at this point in the narrative are removed when they find Jason and are informed by him that, inspired by the influence of Hortense, he has fought off the Great Demon who had tried to destroy him. Further, Jason reveals that he has come to realize in a moment of divine inspiration that Harry is the reincarnated Euripides, Greek playwright and poet, and Hortense, the all-knowing Oracle of Delphi. Before Harry and Hortense leave, Jason passionately kisses Hortense through the bars on the outside window of his room—an important scene to recall when Hortense is later cast as the temptress in Jason's drama.

Using a car jack provided by Harry and Hortense, Jason escapes from Sea Vista and asks Harry and Hortense to meet him at his hideout, an isolated construction site. There he emotionally explains his life and motives as a god. Hortense decides that she must now take action on her belief that Jason desperately needs psychiatric help, and she writes him a letter urging him, as a dear friend, to abandon his fantasies. Among other things, the kiss and the letter serve to cast Hortense as the temptress in Jason's quest. When she and Harry return to Jason to deliver the letter, they discover that he is gone and that a quantity of dynamite has been stolen from the site. Harry and Hortense next encounter Jason as he speaks on the school's PA system, calling for the students to join him in the auditorium to hear his message. There he passionately makes his case to the frenzied mob of students and teachers, while he holds the dean at bay with a wooden board, until finally he is forced to flee, somehow snatching the letter from Hortense as he exits. Soon afterward, Jason dynamites the school's student record room and escapes from the roof using the white-feathered hang glider that Harry and Hortense had seen unfinished in Jason's garage. Powered by a lawn mower motor, he floats away to the cheers of the student body. But the wind currents are too much for him and smash him against the steel girders of a bridge, sending him to his death in the river below.

Alone at the cemetery, Harry and Hortense discover that Jason's boon, "something that the hero wins and brings back so the rest of the world can be better" (148), was the realization "that we were probably all born to be heroes—even the worst of the kids at Hormone High" (149). Harry muses that everyone had lost that awareness and repressed the heroic drive although it was always lying within, waiting for the "ancient magic" to be stirred. Harry resolves that he and Hortense "would always hear the Call to Adventure and . . . would go!" (150), and in that way Jason's boon would be realized.

As is evident from this summary, Paul Zindel has blended elements of the classical heroic quest and the traditional young adult problem novel in structuring this piece. For example, within the framework of the myth of Icarus and Daedalus, he has explored the trauma of parent homicide and parent suicide as they manifest themselves from childhood into young adulthood. All three major characters apparently have no other close school friends and are outside the mainstream in action and thought. That is, in contrast to their hormonal peers, Harry and Hortense are rational, intelligent, caring, independent thinking human beings. Jason's sanity is in question; otherwise he is a kind person. Harry's and Hortense's parents, though virtually nonexistent as characters, are positive adult figures, as are the other adults outside of the school and sanitarium. The school and the sanitarium, as described by Harry, are themselves houses of insanity, or at the least, irrationality. The school, through Harry's eyes, can be seen as a representation of a repressive society unable to grasp the elements of noble character. Harry's vision projects a notion that modern society is a labyrinth mirrored in the minds of its citizens, who are at once monsters and victims too much in the darkness to see that the truth, the key to returning to a more romantic life, is the power of the noble self within themselves. Not only are they unaware of themselves as possible heroes, but unaware that such things as heroes even exist.

A most curious character, in this book of curiosities, is Aunt Mo. She is described by Harry as "a cackling hag" who "had a face with nose capillaries like a road map . . . must have been almost a hundred years old . . . walked . . . doing a little pole vault on a cane . . . wearing tattered army pants and a huge blue sweater . . . her perfume . . . a cross between lilac and atomized bluefish." She also keeps a backyard full of Great Danes and creates "grotesquely inept" paintings of "ancient Guatemalan ceremonial scenes" (26, 27). Later on, while recounting the essential ingredients of a heroic quest, Harry observes, "In almost every story I ever read about a hero, there is always a little old crone or withered man who supplies a gift to help the hero get to where he's got to go" (86). Contextually, this "gift" is the aforementioned car jack. But beyond that is the fact that, aside from Jason's constant companion, Darwin (a black Great Dane), eccentric Aunt Mo's home, for better or worse, has been the only stable force in Jason's life since the death of his parents, a place to recover between horrendous sanitarium and school experiences. Is she representative of, or a distortion of, the "wise old man" archetype?

And then there is Darwin—huge but apparently oblivious to his own potential for terror, destruction, and general mayhem. Should not a creature of this sort in a mythic tale be an evil monster somehow connected to Hades? Appearances deceive. Jason, after all, appears to be the model of the ideal adolescent male but inside is deeply troubled and is destined for self-destruction. Darwin, in spite of his threatening appearance, seems never to have evolved from puppyhood. He is that gentle and vulnerable. Jason finds in Darwin what he is looking for in society: security, unconditional love, and total acceptance. Darwin is Jason to a fault (hubris), innocently consuming the poisoned meat (of the demonic side of school society), but, unlike Jason, saved from death by the teacher and veterinarian (the good side of society in general). There is evil, but also good, and it is so difficult to tell one from the other by appearances alone. One must, like Harry and Hortense and Darwin, simply believe that the goodness is there.

PSYCHOLOGICAL ANALYSIS (Terry M. Pace)

It is apparent that Jason has had little stability in his life and little adult love or guidance. His only reality-based parental figure is his aunt Mo, who appears to be chronically depressed, socially isolated, and like Jason, she may also be delusional. It is not known if Jason witnessed his mother's murder and his father's suicide. But given the tragic yet typical way these events transpire, at age 6 it is very possible that he was in the middle of this terrible scene or was hidden nearby, watching in terror. Murder-suicide tragedies rarely happen to people who have not been disturbed for a long time prior to taking these dramatic steps. Usually there is a history of severe conflict, abuse, and violence in such homes. Most often substance abuse plays a role in the conflict and frequently contributes to the impulsiveness and hopelessness of murder-suicide acts. Frequently, serious depression and anxiety are prominent background factors, and most often there is a multigenerational family pattern of abuse, violence, social maladjustment, lack of achievement, substance abuse, and severe mental illness. It is probable that Jason was also directly abused and suffered emotional neglect in such an environment and that he witnessed many episodes of violence between his parents. When someone like Jason grows up within such an insecure and harsh environment, it is very difficult to develop a secure and stable personal identity (Ainsworth, 1980; Bowlby, 1969, 1973, 1980).

Diagnostically, it is not possible to arrive at a firm assessment of this tragic character. His delusions and sense of social and emotional alienation suggest schizophrenia, and indeed the onset of schizophrenia is commonly encountered during mid- to late adolescence (Beratis, Gabriel, and Hoidas, 1994). However, it is also possible that Jason is not schizophrenic, but suffers from a delusional or psychotic affective-related disorder resulting from his childhood trauma (Campbell et al., 1997; Thompson, 1996; Volkmar, 1996). Either way, the portrayed and implied reality of his life is filled with sadness, meanness, loneliness, rejection, instability, and senseless desperation.

Severely disturbed adolescents usually have disturbed and abusive childhoods, and likewise, severely disturbed adults usually have had painful and unsuccessful experiences during adolescence. One of the most fundamental principles within the science of psychology is the developmental principle, which in general says that previous developmental experiences and processes influence and predict subsequent personal and behavioral outcomes (Ainsworth, 1980; Owens et al., 1995; Robbins and Rutter, 1990; Sroufe, Egelund, and Kreutzer, 1990). That is, what happens in childhood influences who a person is as an adolescent, and what happens during adolescence combines with childhood experiences to influence who a person is as an adult, and so on throughout life. Sadly, Jason experienced nothing but trauma, neglect, rejection, violence, and instability from early childhood through adolescence. Thus, without early and comprehensive intervention, some type of serious impairment or tragic outcome to his life is highly probable, and even with intervention he remains at risk for a variety of continuing social and emotional problems (Eggers and Bunk, 1997; Wolfe and McEachran, 1997).

Whether intervention began when Jason was 6 or at the time we know him in the story at age 16, the basic principles would be the same. Intervention for someone with the problems presented by Jason would be challenging, complex, and long-term in nature. The best intervention plans are founded upon the most sophisticated scientific analysis of the problems the person is presenting with and upon the best research regarding treatment needs and treatment effectiveness (Hibbs and Jensen, 1996; Nathan and Gorman, 1998). At a minimum this involves an appreciation of the complex interactions among the biological, psychological, and social dimensions of human health, and careful, complete, open-minded, professionally critical evaluation and planning for each particular person and situation (Beutler and Clarkin, 1990).

To begin with, the delusional and bizarre symptoms experienced by Jason suggest that he may indeed have a biological illness that renders his brain unable to regulate the activity of the neurotransmitter dopamine and perhaps also serotonin and other neurotransmitters (Kaplan and Sadock, 1998). The major integrative theory about schizophrenia and psychosis is the Diathesis-Stress Model (Kaplan and Sadock, 1998; Nuechterlein et al., 1994). In this model, highly stressful experiences, such as other severe illnesses or psychosocial stress that places exceptional strain on the central nervous system, may serve to activate an underlying genetic vulnerability for schizophrenia.

In the treatment of an adolescent like Jason, one would utilize a multimodal approach (Kopelowicz and Liberman, 1998; McClellan and Werry, 1994). First, a comprehensive evaluation would be needed. This would involve a detailed review of his life and developmental history, medical examination to include neurological studies and mental status assessment, psychological testing to evaluate patterns of cognitive and personality functioning, and a careful review of the appropriateness and safety of his home and school environments. Medication therapy with an antipsychotic agent would serve as a foundation to other treatment efforts. However, medication alone is not enough. First, most people with delusional symptoms are very poor at adhering to prescribed antipsychotic medication. Side effects can be unpleasant and even dangerous, and many people experience paranoid delusions, which makes accepting and understanding the role and importance of medication very difficult. Further, people with schizophrenic and affective symptoms, like Jason, tend to have poor social adjustment and experience instability in living. Lifestyle may be very erratic with little social support and guidance. Thus, even to be successful with medication therapy, social and psychological intervention is required to stabilize emotional and social experiences and provide a consistent and supportive environment.

In most cases, for treatment to be successful, environmental, family, and school intervention are also necessary (Kopelowicz and Liberman, 1998). People, especially children and adolescents, live within social environments where their health and behavior are affected by the stability and dynamics of the people they interact with. For an adolescent, like Jason, neither medication nor psychotherapy are likely to have their maximum benefits unless the daily living and educational environments are structured to be supportive of his needs. From all indications, Jason's aunt is not capable of providing an emotionally stable and safe environment. This would need very careful evaluation. It may be that family and parental, or caretaker, therapy could be of some benefit by helping Jason's aunt to address some of her own emotional and health needs and helping her to provide better guidance and emotional stability for Jason. The emotional environment of the family has been found to be one of the best predictors of relapse in schizophrenic patients and has also been strongly linked to recovery from affective disorders (Falloon et al., 1985; Hogarty et al., 1986). The family is usually taught how to moderate the intensity of emotional expression and maintain a more calm and even emotional climate. Communication skills and practical interpersonal problem-solving skills are provided for all family members. Also, family members are encouraged to develop healthy boundaries between themselves and to decrease overinvolvement in and micromanagement of each other's lives, thus reducing family conflict.

Jason would need to be able to achieve this type of family environment with his aunt or be placed in a setting where such an environment could be provided for him. He may need to be placed in a therapeutic living environment, such as a well-run and well-staffed group home or residential program that included special education resources for his schooling. Successful therapeutic group homes have been developed, but they require significant expertise and resources to operate competently. Effective residential programs are usually modeled after healthy families and communities. Living is family or home based with therapeutic foster parents and a small, carefully matched set of other children. Respect and empathy toward others are taught, and social and personal responsibility are encouraged. There are clear rules for behavior with consistent and appropriate consequences. Positive behaviors are, naturally, rewarded with recognition, appreciation, and access to valued activities. Negative behaviors have a cost, usually loss of freedom to engage in desired activities for a set period of time and the requirement to re-earn access to privileges. Positive communication and social problem-solving skills are actively modeled and taught. In many respects living is otherwise normal, as it might be within a very healthy and adaptable family. Access to specialized psychological and health services is provided for such things as individual counseling and medication.

Whether within an integrated residential-school program or through a separate school, competent special education services would be needed. Such services would need to be based on Jason's individual educational strengths and needs. These needs include his cognitive and intellectual abilities, but it is very important that they also include his emotional and psychological needs. Most school programs for severely emotionally disturbed adolescents provide highly individualized academic instruction, with a practical focus on social and emotional coping and skill development. Such programs, like most residential programs, utilize a structured model of teaching. Clear rules of behavior are established, modeled, practiced, coached, and contingently and consistently reinforced.

Jason's treatment can now be seen as multimodal and interdisciplinary, often involving psychiatrists, psychologists, counselors, social workers, special educators, and therapeutic foster parents. Jason would be provided with a variety of medical, psychological, educational, and environmental treatments, and family intervention is likely to be necessary. Finally, a hallmark of effective treatment of adolescents such as Jason is good case coordination and solid continuity to the treatment team and treatment process (Test, 1992).

Jason's character represents the high-risk adolescent. Without family or emotional stability and with a history of trauma and neglect, Jason faces serious and potentially insurmountable obstacles in his quest for identity and acceptance. There is much to learn from Jason's character, and unfortunately, many adolescents must walk along similarly difficult paths in their own developmental quests. Jason may be understood to be living according to the only thing that has allowed him even a degree of happiness and hope, namely his delusional life of having a loving father and being a well-loved son. Jason's heroism is genuine and represents the heroic struggles of all people to find a sense of security, acceptance, and purpose that gives life positive identity and adaptive meaning. Jason's heroism is not found in his delusional ideas about saving the world, but in his efforts to survive and find a meaningful identity despite the dehumanizing abuse, trauma, rejection, and instability in his life. Jason's delusions are simply the only means available to him in his noble and ultimately human and universal quest for identity and love.

While less dramatic and much more hopeful than Jason's character, the characters of Harry and Hortense are also of psychological interest. The majority of adolescents reading this book would be likely to primarily identify with either Harry or Hortense. These two adolescents are portrayed as high school sweethearts who work together on the school newspaper. Their lives are inseparable. They share almost all their free time and spend hours upon hours talking on the phone with each other at all times of the day and night. Harry and Hortense feel passionately loyal to each other, but this is tinged with doubt and anxiety about the future. They are described as bright and somewhat individualistic kids. Each of them is inquisitive and sensitive with a shared sense of seeking to find adventure and greatness in life. Like many adolescents, they view life from a rather narrow perspective that serves to further their own search for identity and acceptance. The adults in Harry's and Hortense's lives are portrayed as background characters. However, both Harry and Hortense are described as having basically stable and loving families. These characteristics set Harry and Hortense up to pursue their quests for identity and acceptance from very different beginning points and with very different resources than Jason.

Harry is described as an adventuresome and independent kid. He is interested in literature and history, and after reading about Harry Truman, he says he thinks of himself as "give 'em hell Harry," indicating that he does not tolerate disrespect and will not let anything stand in his way when he believes something is the right thing to do. Like that of many adolescents, one of Harry's driving forces is the need to stand his own ground against the tide of adult authority and the status quo. However, also like many adolescents, Harry expresses significant self-doubt and insecurity, and his desire for adventure and greatness leads him to almost become seduced into believing in a literal view of Jason's delusions. Harry's attraction to Jason seems to be based on his overidentification with Jason's dramatic struggles for all the things Harry also wants, namely to make a splash and a difference in the world and to be loved and admired by others. However, the differences between Harry and Jason—their differing family histories—lead Harry to seek his fame by becoming a successful writer, while Jason is doomed to delusional and self-destructive visions.

Hortense's attraction to Jason is based mostly on her identity as a helper or healer. Her life goal is to be a great and famous psychiatrist. Jason's complexity and desperation provide a highly attractive case study for Hortense. However, as often happens to neophyte psychiatrists or psychologists, Hortense begins to feel overwhelmed, frightened, and confused about Jason. She struggles with separation of Jason's needs from her own need to gain self-esteem by helping others. Finally, Hortense and Jason both struggle to understand and control their sexual attraction to each other. The treatment of this theme by the author is very subtle, with only one or two episodes where these sexual tensions are obvious. In the most overt scene, Jason impulsively kisses Hortense through the bars of his room when he is in the sanitarium. Hortense says very little about this event, as if she is embarrassed, confused, or absorbed in thought. Harry experiences jealousy toward Jason and is angry with Hortense for a while after this. These sexual dynamics seem completely normal and predictable for adolescents who are so passionately drawn together.

It is interesting to note the stereotypical nature of Harry's and Hortense's attractions to Jason. Harry's is mostly based on intellectual and adventuresome grounds, while Hortense's attraction is based on her interpersonal compassion and sensitivity as well as some level of sexual attraction for the handsome and charismatic Jason.

As a psychologist, the major concerns I have about Harry and Hortense are with the level of risk they incur when befriending Jason. Basically, their responses to Jason seem healthy and socially admirable. However, as adolescents, their own sense of identity and personal needs are easily confused by their dramatic interactions with Jason. Fortunately, they both come through this experience without harm. However, in real life, many kids are not that lucky. Adolescents are notoriously prone to being attracted by relationships that foster a sense of adventure, rebellion, acceptance, meaning, and identity. However, they often lack the objective judgment to keep themselves out of danger and can be easily swayed by the peer and internal pressures that are inherent. For Hortense, the additional issue of sexual attraction to Jason is also present and must be maturely coped with and resolved.

I have seen many adolescents who appeared to be healthy, normal kids from good and stable families but who simply got in over their heads with attractive yet dangerous types of relationships or activities. The results of such adolescent escapades can be serious and often involve drug or alcohol abuse, unprotected and poorly considered sexual activity, and emotional or physical violence. Drastic consequences can include being physically or sexually abused, having an unplanned pregnancy, acquiring a sexually transmitted disease, developing an alcohol or drug addiction, or becoming an accident victim. Often, long-term depressive and anxiety disorders develop out of these experiences. Problems in school and the propensity for academic failure or dropout increase. Somewhere along the way serious problems develop, and family life becomes unbearable and dysfunctional; the adolescent enters a downward spiral toward poor health and poor social and emotional adjustment.

While both Harry's and Hortense's parents are described as good and loving, they serve as background characters in the book. In real life the best buffer for an adolescent is a loving, stable, emotionally competent family, where some level of joint activity and regular effective communication is maintained with the adolescent without overcontrolling or meddling. While parenting an adolescent is almost always difficult in our times, many parents lack the basic knowledge of adolescent development and the basic relational and communication skills necessary to provide this buffer. There are many professional resources available in almost every community for parenting help. Libraries and bookstores are full of useful guides, and many schools provide information and support for parents, often through the school counselor's office. Psychologists and counselors in private practice and those affiliated with colleges and universities are also important resources to seek out for guidance in parenting today's adolescent.

In Zindel's book, most school officials and teachers are presented in a stereotypical, negative, and incompetent way. While this is sometimes the view of some adolescents, the reality is there are many highly compassionate and professional educators in our school systems. Like parents, educators must work to establish and maintain positive communication with adolescent students. By showing genuine interest in them and treating them with individualized respect, educators may be able to provide critical guidance and buffering for adolescents like Harry and Hortense.

Michael tells me that it is common in young adult literature to tell the story from the adolescent's perspective and to limit adults to minor background characters. While this may make the literature more appealing to the targeted readers, it also portrays a risky view of life. As a psychologist, I can say adolescents most often experience serious troubles whenever there are not loving and responsible adults who are actively, but not excessively, involved in their lives.

It is obvious that Jason did not have parents or other adults who were able to be there for him to the extent he needed. His aunt was too disturbed herself to give Jason the home he needed, even though it seems apparent that she did love him. It also seems that neither the school nor the mental health system provided appropriate adult support for Jason. In school he was treated as a threat and a troublemaker, rather than as a kid with an emotional disability, in need of compassion, understanding, and individualized special education services. In the sanitarium, Jason was treated more as a criminal or an animal who was locked up and medicated into submission. Jason needed and deserved much better than this. He needed the attention of enlightened, respectful, and concerned adults who displayed personalized professionalism.

Harry and Hortense have relatively stable and loving families but are disengaged and alienated from their families and from the adults in their school. Having the stability and love provided in their families is probably the saving grace for Harry and Hortense. However, the lack of communication and openness with their parents or other adults and the high degree of unsupervised independence assumed by Harry and Hortense clearly place them at increased risk for problems. With a more involved and open relationship with their parents or another responsible adult, Harry and Hortense may have been able to talk about their concerns for Jason and their feelings for him. Such open discussion can be a tremendous opportunity for effective guidance and appropriate protection for adolescents.

From a parental or adult point of view, the trick here is to build love, trust, and respect and a habit of open communication with a child from the earliest years onward. Joint activity as a family built around the child's developmental level is essential to this process. Clarity of expectations and consistent, reasonable, nonpunitive discipline is also essential. Parents must then be able to keep up with the development of the child and adolescent and to adapt their involvement, supervision, discipline, and communication to the changing needs and motivations of each child. From my experience as a psychologist and as a parent, I would say these tasks are challenging and difficult, but usually possible. Perfection is not the goal; parents and children will both always make some mistakes. A willingness to learn and a recognition that we are all constantly changing as we age and encounter new stages and issues in our lives are essential.

CONCLUSION

As a psychologist, I think Zindel's book would be a good resource for helping teens discuss and think through many critical concerns encountered while growing up as an adolescent in contemporary America. Parents, teachers, and counselors may also find this book to be of interest, especially as a springboard for discussion of developmental concerns with adolescents or their parents. In *Harry & Hortense at Hormone High*, Paul Zindel captures the spirit of the sometimes lofty, often troubling, and always challenging quest for identity and acceptance during adolescence.

The book explores the heroic quest for identity and acceptance that is central to adolescent experience. Understanding these adolescent characters provides an opportunity for learning about the adolescent search for meaning through the development of individual identity and the pursuit of commitment and acceptance in relationship with others. Also of value is the opportunity to explore the impact of childhood trauma upon adolescent development and the nature of mental illness or severe emotional disturbance. Of special importance to both Michael and me, this book reveals something about the necessary roles of adults in the lives of children and adolescents. Adults—parents, teachers, school administrators, counselors, physicians, and others—are the buffer between emotional disturbance and healthy adjustment, and sometimes even between life and death, for the children and adolescents in their lives. As portrayed by the character of Jason, without the presence and involvement of loving and responsible adults, the risk for tragedy and despair is highly increased.

RECOMMENDED READINGS

Fiction

Burks, Brian. (1995). *Runs with horses*. New York: Harcourt Brace. 118 pp. (ISBN: 0–15–200264–2). MS, HS.

Runs with Horses is a Chiricahua Apache brave who rigorously prepares himself to become a warrior in Geronimo's last band of free Apaches, only to be denied the final test in battle by Geronimo's surrender. For the young brave this historical turn of events is personally traumatic.

Cormier, Robert. (1986). *The chocolate war*. New York: Dell. 191 pp. (ISBN: 0–440–94459–7). HS.

Jerry Renault, a loner in a boys' school, makes decisions that place him at odds with the Vigils, a powerful peer group. He suffers tragic consequences for adhering to his principles. A dark, violent book, but well written and useful.

Crutcher, Chris. (1987). *The crazy horse electric game*. New York: Morrow. 215 pp. (ISBN: 0–688–06683–6). HS.

Willie, a star athlete, finds that his sudden disability tests his relationships with his father and his friends. He discovers his inner strengths and acceptability in another town.

Davis, Terry. (1992). *If rock and roll were a machine*. New York: Delacorte. 209 pp. (ISBN: 0–385–30762–4). MS, HS.

Bert Bowden finds peace in a Harley Davidson road trip, but the journey really is one of self-discovery.

Gallo, Donald. (Ed.). (1997). *No easy answers: Short stories about teenagers making tough choices*. New York: Delacorte. 323 pp. (ISBN: 0–385–32290–9). MS, HS.

The title and subtitle quite reasonably reveal the contents: sixteen short stories that force young protagonists to reach deep and come to terms with personal morals, ethics, and self-identity.

Glenn, Mel. (1997). *Jump ball: A basketball season in poems*. New York: Lodestar. 151 pp. (ISBN: 0–525–67554). MS, HS.

The bus carrying the Tower High School Tigers basketball team overturns on an icy upstate road en route to the state play-offs. The list of injuries and deaths is made more tragic by the reader's intimate knowledge of the life stories of those on the bus: none anticipated the ironies of sudden death and personal loss.

Glenn, Mel. (1997). *The taking of room 114: A hostage drama in poems*. New York: Lodestar. 182 pp. (ISBN: 0–525–67548–5). MS, HS.

A revered high school history teacher snaps and takes his senior history class hostage at gunpoint. Through inner dialogues of character poems, Mel Glenn explores with great delicacy and truth the psyches of students, teachers, members of the extended school community, and the media as they respond to a severe crisis.

Rylant, Cynthia. (1993). *I had seen castles*. New York: Harcourt Brace. 97 pp. (ISBN: 0–15–238003–5). HS.

This is a very powerful novel about love, loss of innocence, and young people in war. It is the dramatic story of one 17-year-old infantryman's loss of the romantic view of war as he endures bodies blown to bits around him day after day during World War II.

Schinto, Jeanne. (Ed.). (1995). *Show me a hero: Contemporary stories about sports*. New York: Persea. 265 pp. (ISBN: 0–89255–209–3). MS, HS.

This extraordinary collection of sports shorts stories pushes the edge of fiction writing. It shoots for the soul of the athlete in all of us: female and male, old and young.

Seabrooke, Brenda. (1997). *Under the pear tree*. New York: Cobblehill. 95 pp. (ISBN: 0–525–65213–2). MS, HS.

Memoir in poetry of the writer's eleventh summer in Fitzgerald, Georgia. A pleasant, uncomplicated poetic read that captures transitions from childhood to young adulthood for several characters.

Nonfiction

Donelson, Kenneth, and Alleen Pace Neilsen. (1989). *Literature for today's young adults*. 3rd ed. Glenview, IL: Scott Foresman. 620 pp. (ISBN: 0–673–47188–8). HS, A.

An extensive resource and bibliography of young adult literature.

Herz, Sarah K., with Donald R. Gallo. (1996). *From Hinton to Hamlet: Building bridges between young adult literature and the classics*. Westport, CT: Greenwood. 144 pp. (ISBN: 0–313–28636–1). A.

An excellent reference text for blending the study of the classics with young adult literature. Excellent practical teaching ideas.

Kaywell, Joan. (1993). *Adolescents at risk: A guide to fiction and nonfiction for young adults, parents, and professionals*. Westport, CT: Greenwood. 288 pp. (ISBN: 0–313–29039–3). HS, A.

A world-class resource for current young adult literature, grouped according to specific social concerns and issues.

Reed, Arthea. (1994). *Reaching Adolescents: The young adult book and the school*. New York: Merrill. 579 pp. (ISBN: 0–023–98861–4). HS, A.

A highly readable and enjoyable introduction to how young adult literature can influence the development of a young adult.

Zvirin, Stephanie. (1992). *The best years of their lives: A resource guide for teenagers in crisis*. Chicago: American Library Association. 122 pp. (ISBN: 0–838–90586–2). HS, A.

A must for teachers who are looking for an easy reference guide to help the students cope with everyday, and some not so everyday, problems.

REFERENCES

Ainsworth, M. S. (1980). Attachment and child abuse. In G. Gerbner, C. J. Ross, and E. Zigler (Eds.), *Child abuse: An agenda for action*, New York: Oxford University Press, 35–47.

Beratis, S., J. Gabriel, and S. Hoidas. (1994). Age at onset in subtypes of schizophrenic disorders. *Schizophrenia Bulletin* 20: 287–296.

Beutler, L. E., and J. F. Clarkin. (1990). *Systematic treatment selection: Toward targeted therapeutic interventions*. New York: Brunner/Mazel.

Bowlby, J. (1969, 1973, 1980). *Attachment and loss*, vols. 1, 2, 3. New York: Basic.

Campbell, M., J. L. Argenteros, E. K. Spencer, S. C. Kowalik, and L. Erlenmeyer-Kimling. (1997). Schizophrenia and psychotic disorders. In J. M. Weiner (Ed.), *Textbook of child and adolescent psychiatry*, 2nd ed. Washington, DC: American Psychiatric Press, 303–332.

Eggers, C., and D. Bunk. (1997). The long-term course of childhood-onset schizophrenia: A 42-year follow-up. *Schizophrenia Bulletin* 23: 117.

Falloon, I. R. H., J. L. Boyd, C. W. McGill, M. Williamson, J. Razani, H. B. Moss, A. M. Gilderman, and G. M. Simpson. (1985). Family management in the prevention of schizophrenia. *Archives of General Psychiatry* 42: 887–896.

Green, A. H. (1997). Physical abuse of children. In J. M. Weiner (Ed.), *Textbook of child and adolescent psychiatry*, 2nd ed. Washington, DC: American Psychiatric Press, 687–697.

Hibbs, E. D., and P. S. Jensen. (Eds.). (1996). *Psychosocial treatments for child and adolescent disorders: Empirically based strategies for clinical practice*. Washington, DC: American Psychological Association.

Hogarty, G. E., C. M. Anderson, D. J. Reiss, S. J. Kornblith, D. P. Greenwald, C. D. Jauna, and M. J. Madonia. (1986). Family education, social skills training and maintenance chemotherapy in aftercare treatment of schizophrenia. *Archives of General Psychiatry* 43: 633–642.

Hogarty, G. E., C. M. Anderson, D. J. Reiss, S. J. Kornblith, D. P. Greenwald, R. F. Ulrich, and M. Carter. (1991). Family psychoeducation, social skills training, and maintenance chemotherapy in the aftercare of schizophrenia, II: Two-year effects of a controlled study on relapse and adjustment. *Archives of General Psychiatry* 48: 340–347.

Kaplan, H. I., and B. J. Sadock. (1998). *Synopsis of psychiatry*, 8th ed. Baltimore: Williams & Wilkins.

Kopelowicz, A., and R. P. Liberman. (1998). Psychosocial treatments for schizophrenia. In P. E. Nathan and J. M. Gorman (Eds.), *A Guide to treatments that work*. New York: Oxford University Press, 190–211.

McClellan, J. M., and J. S. Werry. (1994). Practice parameters for the assessment and treatment of children and adolescents with schizophrenia. *Journal of the American Academy of Child and Adolescent Psychiatry* 33: 616–653.

Mueser, K. T., and H. Berenbaum. (1990). Psychodynamic treatment of schizophrenia: Is there a future? *Psychological Medicine* 20: 253–262.

Nathan, P. E., and J. M. Gorman. (Eds.). (1998). *A Guide to treatments that work*. New York: Oxford University Press.

Nuechterlein, K. H., M. E. Dawson, J. Ventura, M. Gitlin, K. L. Subotnik, K. S. Snyder, J. Mintz, and G. Bartzokis. (1994). The vulnerability/stress model of schizophrenic relapse. *Acta Psychiatrica Scandinavica* 89: 58–64.

Owens, G., J. A. Crowell, H. Pan, D. Treboux, E. O'Conner, and E. Waters. (1995). The prototype hypothesis and the origins of attachment working models: Adult relationships with parent and romantic partners. In E. Waters, B. E. Vaughn, G. Posada, and K. Condo (Eds.), *Caregiving, cultural, and cognitive perspectives on secure base behavior: New growing points of attachment*, monograph of the Society for Research in Child Development 60 (1–2), serial no. 244, pp. 216–233.

Perry, B. D., R. A. Pollard, T. L. Blakley, and D. Vigilante. (1995). Childhood trauma, the neurobiology of adaption, and "use-dependent" development of the brain: How "states" become "traits." *Infant Mental Health Journal* 16: 271–291.

Robbins, L. N., and M. Rutter. (Eds.). (1990). *Straight and devious pathways from childhood to adulthood*. New York: Cambridge University Press.

Sroufe, L. A., B. Egelund, and T. Kreutzer. (1990). The fate of early experience following developmental change: Longitudinal approaches to individual adaption in childhood. *Child Development* 61: 1363–1373.

Test, M. A. (1992). Training in community living. In R. P. Liberman (Ed.), *Handbook of psychiatric rehabilitation*. New York: Macmillan, 153–170.

Thompson, P. H. (1996). Schizophrenia with childhood and adolescent onset—a nationwide register-based study. *Acta Psychiatrica Scandinavica* 94: 187–193.

Volkmar, F. R. (1996). Childhood and adolescent psychosis: A review of the past 10 years. *Journal of the American Academy of Child and Adolescent Psychiatry* 35: 843–851.

Wolfe, D. A., and A. McEachran. (1997). Child physical abuse and neglect. In E. J. Mash and L. G. Terdal (Eds.), *Assessment of childhood disorders*, 3rd ed. New York: Guilford, 523–568.

Wolfe, D. A., and C. Wekerle. (1993). Treatment strategies for child physical abuse and neglect: A critical report. *Clinical Psychological Review* 13: 473–500.

Zindel, P. (1984). *Harry & Hortense at Hormone High*. New York: Harper and Row.

Index

ment avoiding, 46; help damaging, 43–44; identity assistance, 47–48; individuation development, 44; mental health stigma, 43; parental attitudes, 45; peer group role, 44; PFLAG, 49; religion vs. sexual orientation, 46–47; sexual identity help, 47–48; stereotype relevance, 47; treatment alternatives, 44

Homosexuality: attitude indicators, 50; counseling help, 47–48; family rejection fears, 40; gay men vs. lesbian attitudes, 47; hate crimes against, 40; school role, 49–50; society attitude changes, 40–41; suicide rates, 40; verbal labeling of, 39–40. *See also* Sexual identity

Identity confusion: book character development, 132–135; book synopsis, 130–132; cognitive development, 133–134; conclusions on, 136–137; identity formation, 136; introduction to, 129–130; physical development, 133; puberty changes, 129; social development, 135

Identity development: identity crisis, 7; parental involvement, 146–147; process of, 146

Identity formation: gender identity and, 136; vs. identity confusion, 136

Identity searching: adolescent tasks in, 171–172; anger manifestations, 172; family crisis, 172; moral identity and, 171–172; process of, 171

Imago Relationship Therapy: content of, 82; family observations, 83; intentional vs. reactive relationships, 82; life partner choice, 82; original purpose, 82; parent-child vs. adult

relationships, 83; parenting premise, 82

Industry: normative crisis resolution, 13; psychological growth, 13; vs. inferiority, 13

Initiative, vs. guilt, 12

Integrity, sexual minority organization, 52

Intimacy: book analysis, 62; book synopsis, 60–62; conclusions, 68; counseling for, 63–67; domestic violence and, 59; emotional connectedness locations, 60; identity questions for, 59–60; introduction, 59–60; positive models for, 59; therapy for, 63–67

Intimacy analysis: book messages, 62; girls identifying with, 62

Intimacy therapy: abusive relationship recognizing, 67; boy's relationship knowledge, 67; Erikson's adolescent period, 65–66; intimacy reasons for, 66–67; parent and teen relationships, 63–64; self development, 64; sex vs. friendship, 65; stereotyping perpetuating, 64

Jewish prejudice. *See* Prejudice realizations

Lesbian women. *See* Homosexuality

Marcia, James, 7

Maslow, Abraham, 113

Men: body image and success, 23. *See also* Father-son relationships; Father-son therapy

Metropolitan Community Church, 52

Metropolitan Life Insurance Company, 24

Nabozny, Jeremy, 51

Needs meeting: gang activities and,

About the Contributors

LYNNE B. ALVINE is associate professor and coordinator of the Master of Arts in Teaching English Program at Indiana University of Pennsylvania. A former middle and high school English teacher, she is now a nationally recognized educational researcher and lecturer in English education.

MICHAEL L. ANGELOTTI is professor of education at the University of Oklahoma, Norman. An accomplished teacher and writer, he is editor of *English International*, director of the Oklahoma Writing Project, and poet in residence for the Oklahoma Arts Council.

JOAN BAUER is the author of *Squashed*, winner of the Delacorte Press Prize for a First Young Adult Novel and the School Library Journal Best Book of the Year Award. Her other novels include *Thwonk*, an American Library Association Top Ten Best Book for Young Adults, *Rules of the Road* (Putnam), and *Sticks*.

PATRICIA A. CRAWFORD is assistant professor of reading and language arts education at the University of Central Florida, Orlando. A former elementary teacher, her writing appears in *Language Arts, Teaching and Learning Literature, The New Advocate*, and *The Journal of Research in Childhood Education*.

DAVID B. DANIEL is assistant professor of psychology at the University of Maine, Farmington. A specialist in child and adolescent development, he has worked in a variety of settings, most notably an Indian reservation and a group home.

PATRICIA L. DANIEL is assistant professor of English education at the University of South Florida, Tampa. Her writings have appeared in *English Journal, Language Arts, Equity and Excellence in Education*, and *Adolescent Literature as a Complement to the Classics*, volumes 1 and 2 (Christopher-Gordon), and *Using Literature to Help Troubled Teenagers Cope with Family Issues* (Greenwood).

RITA G. DRAPKIN is associate professor and assistant director of counseling and student development at Indiana University of Pennsylvania. She is a licensed psychologist and provides individual and group psychotherapy at the university and in private practice.

CHARLES R. DUKE is dean of the Reich College of Education and professor of reading at Appalachian State University in Boone, North Carolina. He has published numerous articles about teaching and education, and has authored five books. His latest work is *Poets' Perspectives: Reading, Writing and Teaching Poetry* (Heinemann, 1992).

JESSANNA (TANNA) M. GARTSIDE is a former guidance counselor with the Volusia County School System, Daytona Beach, Florida. Her specialty is developing parental support groups to help with conflict resolution.

MARGARET GOLDMAN is a practicing attorney in Tempe, Arizona. She is the founder of Care Comix, a national acquaintance rape program, and Barriers Down, a respect and rape prevention education program.

MARIE HARDENBROOK is a school librarian for the Tempe, Arizona, School System. She is currently a doctoral student in curriculum and instruction at Arizona State University, Tempe.

J. ROY HOPKINS is professor of psychology at St. Mary's College of Maryland. He has written extensively in the field of psychology, most notably *Adolescence: The Transitional Years* and a coauthored introductory textbook titled *Psychology*.

JEFFREY S. KAPLAN is assistant professor of educational foundations at the University of Central Florida, Daytona Beach. His publications include articles in *English Journal, School Counselor, The ALAN Review*, and chapters in *United in Diversity* (National Council of Teachers of English), *Adolescent Literature as a Complement to the Classics* (Christopher-Gordon), and *Using Literature to Help Troubled Teenagers Cope with Family Issues* (Greenwood).

JANET E. KAUFMAN is assistant professor of English at the University of Utah, Provo. A former middle and high school teacher, her specialty is multicultural literature and pedagogy that emphasizes the emotional life of students.

LYNN KAUFMAN is a social worker at the Kew Valley Center in Kansas City, Kansas, and an adjunct instructor at the University of Kansas School of Social Welfare. She is responsible for individual and group therapy for Kew Valley's preadolescents.

JENNIFER KHERA is cofounder of Barriers Down in Tempe, Arizona. Barriers Down is an educational program to help teenagers deal with questions of rape.

MARY E. LITTLE is assistant professor of special education at the University of Central Florida, Daytona Beach. An accomplished consultant and lecturer, her recent research is on the impact of professional development schools on teacher education practices.

PATTI MAHONEY is a mental health counselor in private practice in Tempe, Arizona. For sixteen years, she was a middle and high school teacher in Arizona.

VICKI J. McENTIRE is the clinical manager of the acute care services of the Harbor Behavioral Health Care Institute in New Port Richey, Florida. Her specialty is crisis intervention and counseling, and she has worked extensively in communities throughout the United States.

MARY ALICE MEYERS is a school psychologist for Volusia County Schools, Daytona Beach, Florida. Her responsibilities include providing psychological evaluations and developing appropriate academic and behavioral interventions.

MARCIA F. NASH is professor of literacy education at the University of Maine, Farmington. A respected teacher and lecturer, she has contributed to many journals and has served as the coeditor of a book review column for *Language Arts*.

TERRY M. PACE is associate professor of counseling psychology at the University of Oklahoma, Norman. A licensed psychologist, he is director of the University of Oklahoma Psychology Clinic.

KRISTEN STERNBERG is the technology consultant for the Dalton School, New York City. She holds a master's degree in exceptional education from the University of Central Florida and is interested in integrating her background in computer science with her love for music.

LOIS T. STOVER is professor of education and chair of the Educational Studies Department at St. Mary's College of Maryland. Her books include *Creating Interactive Environments in Secondary Schools* (with Gloria Neubert and Jim Lawlor), *Presenting Phyllis Reynolds Naylor*, and *Young Adult Literature: The Heart of the Middle School Curriculum*.

ROSARIA C. UPCHURCH is a licensed marriage and family therapist with an office in Daytona Beach, Florida. She operates a general practice and presents training workshops in human growth and development.

JON L. WINEK is assistant professor and coordinator of the Marriage and Family Therapy Program in the Department of Psychological Counseling at Appalachian State University in Boone, North Carolina. He is a clinical member and approved supervisor in the American Association for Marriage and Family Therapy.